the
beauty
battle

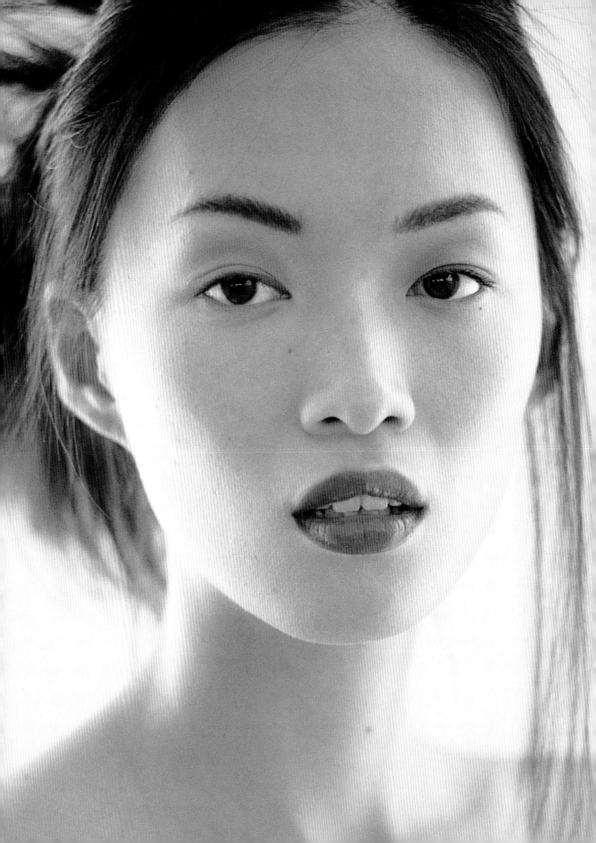

Wendy Lewis

the beauty battle

the insider's guide to wrinkle rescue and cosmetic perfection from head to toe

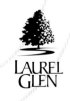

LAUREL
GLEN

San Diego, California

Laurel Glen Publishing

An imprint of the Advantage Publishers Group

5880 Oberlin Drive, San Diego, CA 92121-4794

www.laurelglenbooks.com

All notations of errors or omissions should be addressed to Laurel Glen Publishing, Editorial Department, at the above address. All other correspondence (author inquiries, permissions, and rights) concerning the content of this book should be addressed to Quadrille Publishing, Alhambra House, 27–31 Charing Cross Rd., London WC2H 025, England.

ISBN 1-59223-029-6

Library of Congress Cataloging-in-Publication Data available upon request.

Printed in Singapore

1 2 3 4 5   07 06 05 04 03

Editorial Director: **Jane O'Shea**

Creative Director: **Mary Evans**

Designer: **Sue Storey**

Project Editor: **Lisa Pendreigh**

Editor: **Katie Ginn**

Picture Research: **Nadine Bazar**

Illustrations: **Sue Storey**

Production: **Nancy Roberts and Beverley Richardson**

Contents

The three major advances in the arena of beauty treatments and aesthetic medicine in recent years—botulinum toxin, liposuction, and lasers—have become mainstream because they are safe, effective, predictable, and can forestall surgical intervention. For more than ten years, Wendy Lewis has been consulting with hundreds of clients, each in search of advice as they consider cosmetic surgery and other alternatives. Here she has distilled her vast knowledge of the aging complexion, hair, body, and the onset of dreaded wrinkles, so that all women can arm themselves with crucial insider information previously available only to her inside circle in New York and London.

Short of surgery, peels, and beauty shots, the best thing a woman can do to slow down the inevitable appearance of wrinkles is to start the prevention process early—like yesterday. Start practicing good skin habits while your crow's-feet are still fine lines, and you should be able to stay wrinkle-free for a whole lot longer. Wrinkles are basically folds of the skin that multiply with age and are most common on the face and hands. Skin thickness varies according to body area, and the epidermis thins as time goes by, especially in thin-skinned regions such as around the eyes and neck. The sun is Public Enemy #1 when it comes to the complexion changes we see with age. Smoking is Public Enemy #2, alcohol is #3, and next on the list is poor nutrition. Sunscreen protection is mandatory, as photoaging is sure to speed up the hands of your aging clock. After thirty, skin becomes pale, sallow, muddy, and dull for three reasons: The blood supply to the skin gets sluggish, the shedding of dead cells generally slows, and cells regenerate at different rates, causing uneven pigmentation, lines, age spots, and a dried-out, leathery surface.

With the marketplace so flooded, it's easy to get confused by the science and advertising of cosmeceuticals today. In addition to smart prevention and maintenance tips, Wendy shares the latest scoop on the most state-of-the-art solutions science has to offer, and the informed distinction between what works and what's a waste of your time and money. The cornerstone product that I start all my patients on is Retin-A cream, which works for wrinkles as well as acne. In several months of continuous use, your skin can look more uniform in color and texture; fine lines soften and brown spots fade.

And getting your beauty sleep is not a myth either. Night is a time when your body slows down to repair itself and your skin needs nourishment to counteract the effects of environmental abuse. The latest formulas contain potent antioxidants, growth factors, and megavitamins to replenish and rejuvenate. Technology is developing to keep us just about wrinkle- and fat-free, with glowing skin, a flawless body, and a full head of beautiful hair forever. It's just a matter of time.

Seth Matarasso, M.D., Associate Clinical Professor of Dermatology at the University of California, San Francisco, School of Medicine

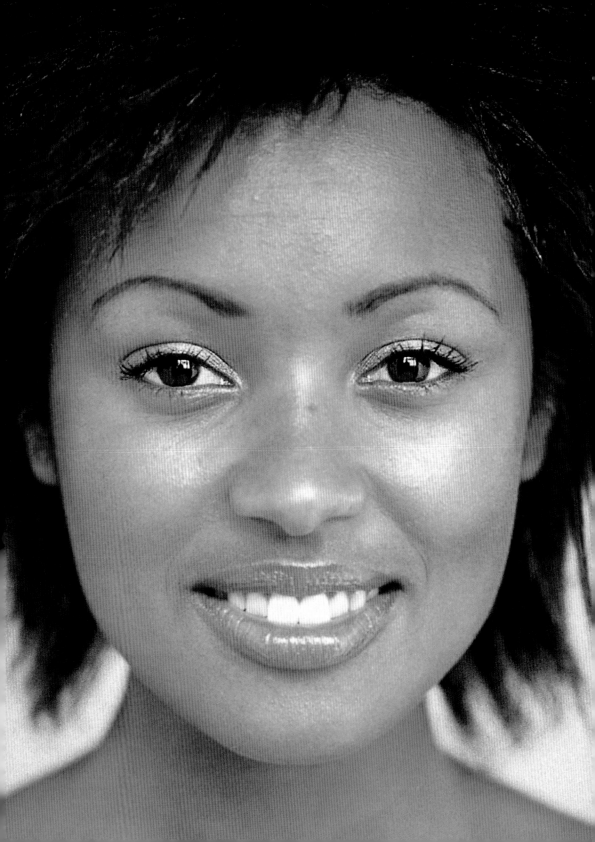

COMPLEXION PERFECTION

Hormonal and other internal upheavals have a way of leaving their mark on your skin, in the form of skin eruptions and other lumps and bumps. Acne is the most common skin disease, but only 7 percent of the 70 million sufferers ever see a dermatologist for help. Acne is a buildup of dried oil and dead skin cells in the hair follicles under the skin. Hormones, particularly male hormones called androgens, stimulate the hormone-sensitive sebaceous glands, which produce sebum. As with many other skin conditions, genetics plays a part. All of these factors work together to start the vicious acne cycle.

If bad skin is a major problem in your life, join the club. The occasional pimple is to be expected—we all have oil glands and sometimes they get clogged. The good news is that help is at hand. Whether you have an occasional flare-up or chronic acne that makes you want to hide, there are many effective treatment options. There's still no cure, with or without a prescription. The secret to controlling it is PREVENTION. Most acne therapies require ongoing treatment to keep your skin clear. Even after blemishes disappear, using an effective acne treatment will keep new ones from forming. The first step is determining the type and cause of your acne.

demystifying pimples

Pimples come in a variety of forms, but they all start out the same—as a plugged-up follicle. They actually begin two to three weeks before the blemishes show up on your face.

Blackheads are formed when dead skin cells and sebum are packed inside a follicle where the walls have broken. If the plug enlarges and pops out of the duct, it's a blackhead.

Whiteheads are formed on or under the skin, showing up as a skin-colored or inflamed bump. The opening of the plugged sebaceous follicle is closed or very narrow, instead of open. With inflammatory acne, whiteheads become infected with bacteria, causing them to swell.

Papules are red, raised bumps or inflamed lesions that occur when oily materials inside the follicle rupture into the skin. They show up as small, solid lesions, slightly elevated above the surface of the skin.

Pustules are dome-shaped lesions similar to papules but inflamed with pus. Pustules formed over sebaceous follicles usually have a hair in the center. Pustules that heal without turning into a cystic form don't usually scar.

Cysts are a severe form of inflammatory acne—closed, hard sacs that can be large and painful. A cyst extends into the deep layers of the skin where they can destroy tissue structures and cause scarring.

spotting causes

Acne is often linked to genetics and stress. Adding hormones to the mix can really defeat your skin. Getting to the root of the problem can be a challenge.

Hormones—specifically androgens produced by the ovaries and adrenal glands in women—trigger most acne attacks. Androgens cause sebaceous glands to enlarge; when they get overstimulated, acne flares up. Acne can crop up any time hormones are in flux—during puberty, pregnancy, or menopause. A few pimples showing up every month is not necessarily acne.

Oil production increases as sebaceous glands are stimulated by androgens; oil accumulates in the follicle and travels up hair shafts to the skin's surface. As it travels, it mixes with bacteria and dead skin cells shed from the lining of the follicle. The greater the oil production, the greater the likelihood that the hair follicle will become clogged and result in an eruption.

Follicle changes occur as androgen levels increase and sebaceous glands enlarge. Normally, dead cells inside the follicle are expelled onto the surface. During hormonal flux, these cells are shed more rapidly and stick together. When mixed with sebum, they clog the follicle and form a plug.

Bacteria breeds wildly in clogged sebaceous glands and follicles. *Propionibacterium acnes (P. acnes)* multiply rapidly and chemicals produced by the bacteria can cause inflammation in the follicle and surrounding skin.

raging hormones

Once you've survived the awkward teenage years—wearing braces, studying for exams, and taking bad school photos—you would expect to have left problem skin behind.

Teens with bad complexions are often told things like "Don't worry, lots of kids your age go through this," or "You'll grow out of it." While millions of teenagers suffer before emerging clear-skinned, others are not so fortunate. Sometimes your skin doesn't clear up after you finish high school. Acne may not even start until adulthood. Perhaps you sailed through your teens with perfect skin, only to start breaking out in your twenties, thirties, or forties.

REALITY CHECK: Oily skin tends to develop lines and wrinkles at a slower rate, so your oily skin may actually be keeping your skin looking younger for longer.

A staggering four million adults worldwide suffer from acne. Many cases begin in adulthood, often accompanying the hormonal changes of pregnancy, irregularities in the menstrual cycle, or ovarian cysts, which may increase androgen productivity. Women typically suffer from adult onset or worsening acne more often than men, and they may have the problem for many years. Stress almost always plays a role because it stimulates the gland that produces androgens. When you feel stressed, your hormone levels fluctuate, which can cause increased oil production in the skin. Most of us notice an extra blemish or two before a major event in our lives.

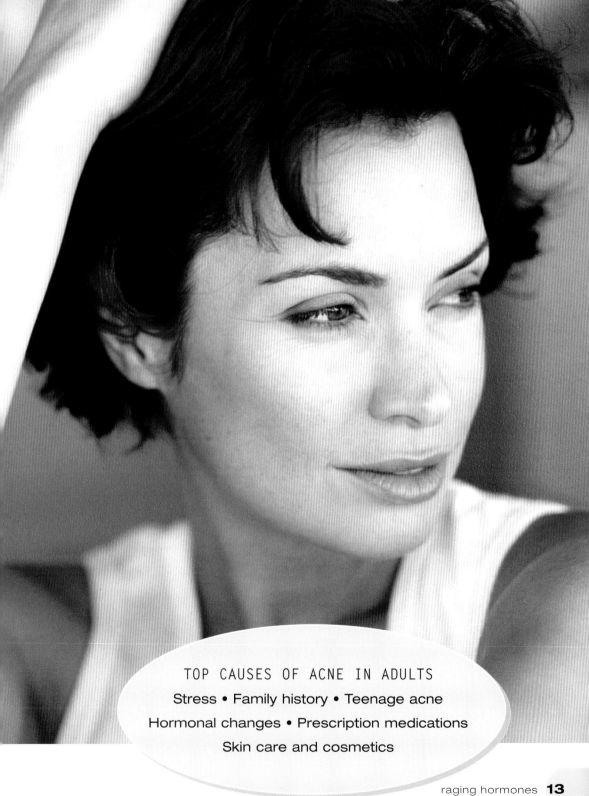

TOP CAUSES OF ACNE IN ADULTS
Stress • Family history • Teenage acne
Hormonal changes • Prescription medications
Skin care and cosmetics

acne cycle

It's that time of the month. Many women experience monthly outbreaks caused by the release of progesterone after ovulation.

Hormonal medications and endocrine disorders are cited as causes of acne flare-ups in grown women. Even slight hormonal fluctuations can increase the number of new pimples, blackheads, and whiteheads, as well as the oiliness of the forehead and cheeks. This is most common at about five days before the beginning of the cycle and continues for seven to ten days. You should adjust your skin-care regime to account for these monthly fluctuations.

Some women are genetically prone to drastic hormone swings, higher levels of androgens, and oil glands that are more sensitive to hormones. Your doctor may recommend taking an oral contraceptive to change the balance between androgenic and female hormones and help control acne breakouts. Oral contraceptives change your hormone levels, and can cause breakouts both when started and stopped. Some birth control pills are specially formulated to control acne, and Ortho Tri-Cyclen has been approved by the Food and Drug Administration (FDA) for the treatment of acne. This pill treats acne with a combination of ethinyl estradiol, a synthetic estrogen, and norgestimate, a progestin. Although the oral contraceptive that has been studied clinically with regard to acne is Ortho Tri-Cyclen, many dermatologists believe that any formulation with a low amount of androgen can be used to treat acne. The pill may not be effective at all, or only for a certain period of time. For some lucky women, it can be the answer to their acne woes. Improvement doesn't necessarily mean an end to complexion worries, but for some women, if their acne is better than it was, they're happy. The pill can be combined with other standard acne treatments like retinoids and antibiotics for maximum effectiveness. If your acne gets worse, other therapies will be needed. When bacteria enter into the picture and inflammation and redness become evident, more aggressive treatments such as oral antibiotics may be necessary. The pill can also have side effects, including weight gain, blood clots, heart attack, stroke, hypertension, and diabetes. These risks are higher in women who smoke, and increase with age.

Your gynecologist might suggest blood tests or an ultrasound to pinpoint any underlying hormonal imbalances that could be a contributing cause to your acne. Irregular periods, excess facial hair, oily skin, and acne may be a sign of polycystic ovarian syndrome (PCOS), in which excess production of androgenic hormones may lead to these conditions. When in doubt seek the help of a doctor.

BEAUTY BYTES:

For information on oral contraceptives, go to www.orthotricyclen.com.

teen troubles

When your skin is breaking out and turns on the shine, you feel like you just want to hide. Your best bet is to take the fast track to oil control.

- Do you have blackheads? Get a vitamin A derivative, like retinoic acid, to get deep into oil plugs and stop the clog.

- Don't overdo topical acne medications—use only a thin layer. They can dry out your skin.

- If you can feel hard lumps deep under the skin, see a dermatologist. Don't self-treat.

- Less is more. Be careful not to scrub, massage, or cleanse excessively.

- Don't touch your face more than you absolutely have to. Hands can spread bacteria.

- Don't get discouraged if a treatment isn't working. Seek advice about switching to something that may be more effective.

- Once you find that magic combination that keeps your acne under control, stick with it.

- Work to keep skin balanced—a good ratio of oily to dry. Be careful not to overdo it with drying formulas that leave skin raw and red. Oily skin may not need a moisturizer every day, especially in warm weather and humidity.

pregnant pores

If you have a history of acne, your skin may either improve or get worse when you are expecting a child. Acne can appear at any stage during pregnancy and may or may not clear up on its own after childbirth.

When you're pregnant, anything goes. You can break out on the face, chest, back, or elsewhere. Random flare-ups can happen at any time, especially in the first trimester, and may ease up during the second. Although prenatal acne cannot be prevented, there are steps you can take to minimize breakouts. Keep your skin in good shape before and after becoming pregnant and practice early intervention. Keep it simple—during pregnancy, skin reactivity changes a lot and your skin may be sensitive to certain ingredients. Some glycolic acid products are considered safe for use by pregnant women, but most common acne treatments are a no-no—whatever is done to the mother may affect the fetus. Medications like antibiotics, vitamin A derivatives, and benzoyl peroxide should not be used by pregnant women or resumed until the baby is weaned. Salicylic acid is not generally recommended, as it is absorbed through the skin and can interfere with blood clotting. These drugs fall under the FDA "Pregnancy Category C," meaning that animal studies have not been conducted and it is unknown whether they can harm the fetus or if the drug is excreted in human milk. The final decision should always be left to your obstetrician or pediatrician.

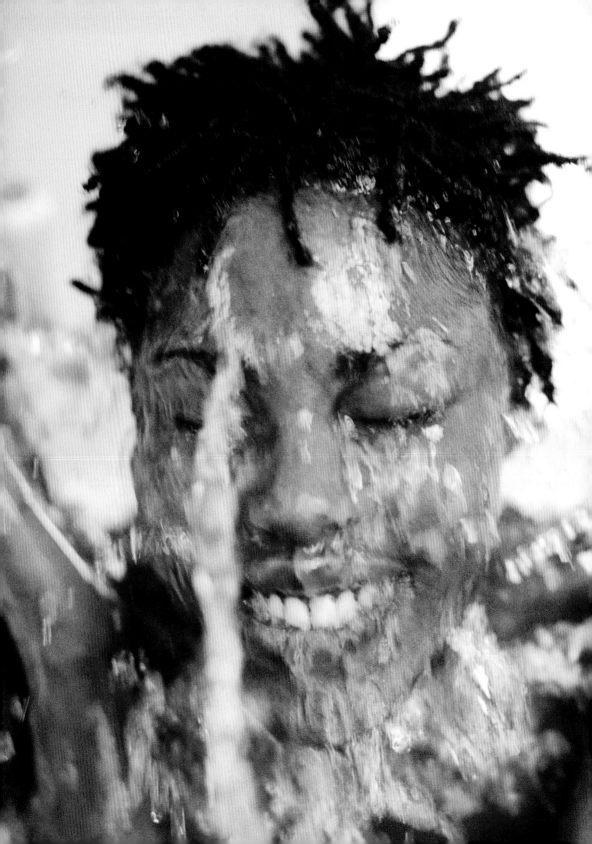

OIL PATROL

Forget what you've been hearing for ages. The secret to reducing your shine lies more in what you put on your skin than what you put into your body. Contrary to popular myth, controlling oil glands is not food related, so following a strictly no-grease diet won't clear your skin. (While gorging on french fries, chocolate, and other greasy foods may not cause acne, it won't do wonders for the way your clothes fit.) Drinking lots of water won't really help acne either, even though it is good for you in other ways.

As with all things skin related, do what works for you. A few foods could present a problem. Some women swear they break out after consuming chocolate, ketchup, or soda. Avoiding allergenic substances such as dairy, caffeine, and alcohol is sometimes recommended. Excessive iodine, found in fast foods, milk, and shellfish, has been cited as an acne trigger. If there might be a connection, it would be prudent to avoid those foods that seem to aggravate pimples. No one knows your skin like you do.

The same applies to skin care products. The trick is to eliminate excess shine without stripping the skin of its natural oils, and to avoid overuse and incorrect application of the formulas that can help control your acne. Don't smother your skin with your acne products or paint them on heavily like a mask.

squeaky clean

You can't scrub pimples away. Cleansing overload can aggravate skin and slow down the healing process. The key to good cleansing is using the right products.

Work gently to unclog pores of oil and fight the bacteria that cause the microinfection that turns into acne. It is natural to want to overcleanse and overexfoliate to wage war on every last drop of oil in the skin. This can trigger breakouts, as your oil glands will overcompensate. Acne doesn't necessarily mean your face is dirty. If you aren't washing thoroughly enough, dirt can clog pores and cause pimples, but if you are constantly stripping away essential oils that your skin can't replace, you may be drying out the surface layer and making your skin less able to hold its own moisture. If your skin is dry, it will produce more oil, which is more likely to become trapped in your pores.

Don't use soap that can dry out the skin. Wash gently with a small amount of soap-free, scent-free cleanser. Wash your face from under the jaw to the hairline. Thoroughly rinse to get rid of any film from the cleanser. Astringents should be used only on oily areas. If your skin gets shiny or doesn't feel clean without an astringent, stick to alcohol-free, soothing toners. Abrasive cleansers and harsh exfoliants can aggravate acne. Gentle exfoliating cleansers with micro-particle-sized beads can work to get the gunk out and dislodge blackheads.

TOP TIP:
Always use a fresh washcloth to avoid bacteria that can grow in damp fabric.

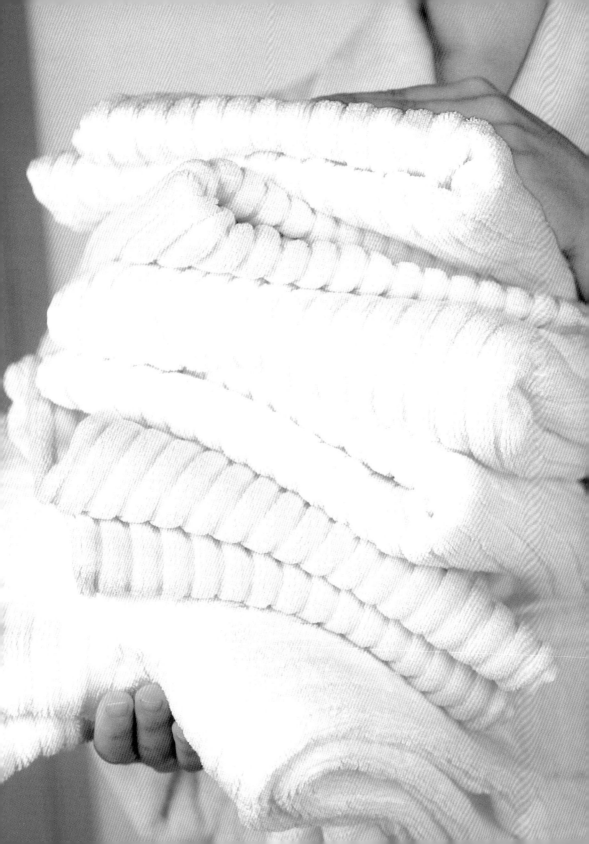

balancing act

Acne and dry skin can coexist on the same face. Acne treatments can be very drying, especially if you have dry skin or eczema to start with. The key is to strike a balance.

Dry skin indicates that it is lacking oil, whereas dehydrated skin means a lack of water. Oily skin can be dehydrated even though it has plenty of oil. If you attempt to strip skin of all its oil content, you may end up with skin that is even oilier. Try a gentle, noncreamy cleanser and an oil-free moisturizing product. Look for words like "mild," "nonirritating," and "nondrying." Be careful with cleansers that contain medications like salicylic acid. For best results, cleanse first and then apply your medication so you don't layer up, which can add to irritation.

The "T-zone" runs from the forehead down the nose to the chin, where oil glands are most plentiful. Some surface grease on the skin is normal—it has the job of lubricating the skin's outer layer and keeping it protected. Most people who suffer from excess grease see the bulk of it on the forehead and nose, the most common locations for acne. Humidity and high temperatures can wreak havoc on your T-zone as well, leaving it shiny. If you're active and enjoy sports, perspiration may add to your shine.

Purging your pores of surface oil and debris will keep them open, which translates into making them look tighter. The thicker and oilier your skin, the larger and more noticeable your pores will be. Shine also draws attention to pore size.

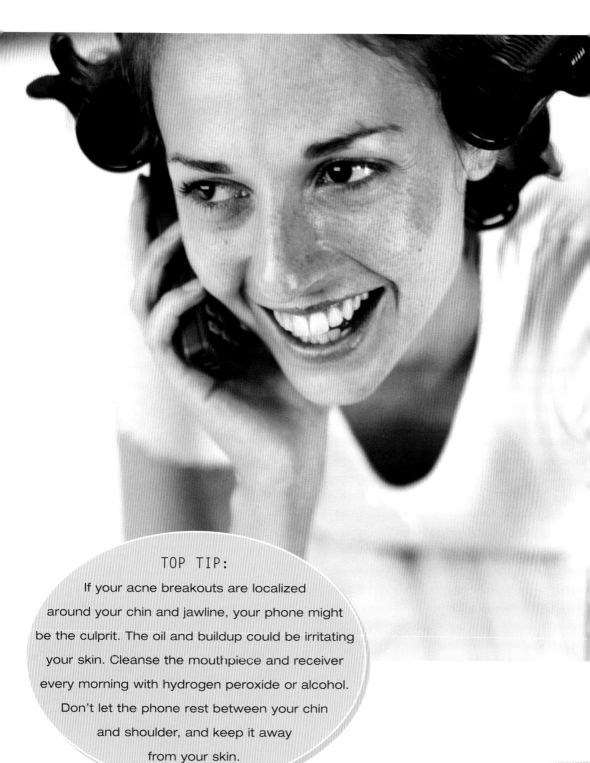

TOP TIP:

If your acne breakouts are localized around your chin and jawline, your phone might be the culprit. The oil and buildup could be irritating your skin. Cleanse the mouthpiece and receiver every morning with hydrogen peroxide or alcohol. Don't let the phone rest between your chin and shoulder, and keep it away from your skin.

tackling outbreaks

Your first course of action is to treat skin eruptions on your own. Start by reviewing what you are currently using. Your skin-care regime may actually be the culprit.

More women are seeking anti-acne treatments than ever before. We seem to have an insatiable appetite for new and improved treatments, both prescription and over-the-counter varieties. Every acne sufferer has encountered over-the-counter products that only work for a short time.

Choose products specially designed for oily skin types that won't clog pores. Blotting out the oil, soaking it up, and keeping skin shine-free can be a full-time job. Many moisturizers, creams, and other skin-care and cosmetic products contain fats, oils, and waxes that can clog pores and make problem skin worse. Whatever you do, declare a moratorium on any product that feels creamy, heavy, or isn't oil-free. Women who are nearing forty may feel inclined to focus on moisturization and as a result, overload their skin with pore-clogging ingredients such as lanolin, cocoa butter, sesame oil, and avocado oil. Gels or lighter lotions are better suited to oily skin.

Pore size is genetically determined. Nothing has been proved to permanently shrink them. Keeping pores clean and unplugged can make them look smaller. Pore strips may help, but they really can't go deep enough to extract the gunk that's buried. You can prevent the keratinized plug from forming with good exfoliation. Masks that contain kaolin, calamine, or clay can absorb excess oil, calm the skin, and keep pores toned.

Exfoliation is very important when it comes to caring for oily, acne-prone skin. First, figure out if your skin thickness is thin, medium, or thick by judging its strength, resiliency, and general condition. Healthy skin is smooth, firm, tight, even, and has good tolerance levels. If your skin is fragile, you need to increase skin thickness by stimulating new collagen, which is what Retin-A does. Thick skin needs to be well exfoliated to keep its barrier function intact. Look for more active concentrations of alpha hydroxy acid (AHA), or glycolic and lactic acid, and beta hydroxy acid (BHA), or salicylic acid, to produce a superficial glow and keep pores unclogged. If your skin can tolerate higher concentrations, it will clear up faster.

Women with acne often need to switch from some of the cosmetics they use to oil-free formulas. Lip products that contain moisturizers may cause small open and closed comedos to form. Hairstyling products that come into contact with the skin along the hairline can cause burning or stinging in people with acne. Hair dyes that contain coal tar have been cited as potential triggers. Other lesser-known irritants include fabric softeners, perfume, and hair spray. Choose formulas that are nonacnegenic (won't cause acne, pustules, or papules) and noncomedogenic (won't cause comedos, like blackheads or whiteheads). Some women find that even products labeled as noncomedogenic may cause acne.

> **TOP TIP:**
> An oil-free product can become oil based when it comes into contact with the natural oils in your skin and environmental debris.

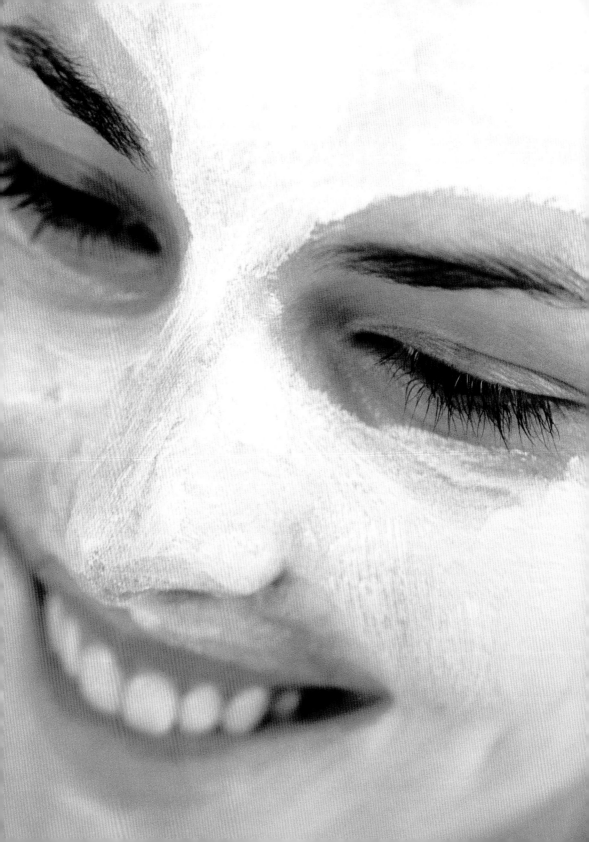

dos and don'ts for perfect skin

- **DO** wash skin with a mild, detergent-free cleanser that doesn't leave a residue.

- **DO** use a clay-based mask treatment once a week to eliminate excess oiliness.

- **DO** treat your skin to a series of superficial peels to clean out pores.

- **DO** avoid rough scrubbing and massage, which can stimulate glands.

- **DON'T** pick or squeeze pimples. This can spread infection, delay healing, and cause long-term scarring.

- **DO** rinse with cold water after cleansing and use an alcohol-free toner.

- **DO** use a fresh washcloth daily to avoid bacteria that can grow in damp fabric.

- **DO** shampoo hair daily and avoid heavy conditioners, and don't let your hair hang over your face.

- **DON'T** give up too soon. Give therapies at least six weeks to kick in.

- **DO** wash your face after exercising to remove sweat and dirt.

- **DO** stop touching your face to avoid spreading the bacteria that cause acne.

- **DO** use oil-free sunscreen with SPF 15, titanium dioxide, and micronized zinc.

buffed up

If you suffer from acne, choose your skin specialist wisely. Not all therapists are trained in the accurate assessment of problem skin and its special needs.

All acne treatments should be given under sanitary conditions to provide the most healing results. Mild steam cleansing together with an exfoliation treatment to remove dead topical cells, extractions, and a soothing, healing mask is the best course. Facial scrubs that buff away excess oil, dirt, and dead skin can also give skin a big boost. However, rubbing and massaging can cause irritation, and intense facial massage, rich European-style facial creams, and overhandling of delicate pores can aggravate acne and cause eruptions. If your skin looks like it went through a war after a facial treatment, your technician may be too heavy-handed and aggressive.

Whiteheads are closed comedos and should only be extracted in the hands of an expert. A dermatologist may use a sterile needle to prick the tip of the pimple—do not try this at home. When you squeeze them yourself, you risk making the situation worse. As an alternative, try applying a salicylic gel or cream to help unplug the pore. Holding ice to the area whenever you feel the urge to touch it can help.

Milia are deep little white bumps that form like tiny cysts. Exfoliation can help get rid of them by unroofing the skin cells that are trapped and sloughing them away.

do-it-yourself facial

- **Cleansing:** Apply a cleanser with the fingertips and work into the skin. Remove completely with a washcloth.

- **Steaming:** Apply a warm washcloth to the face to soften the skin and relax pores.

- **Extraction:** With a soft paper tissue around your two fingers, gently squeeze the pore. If the oil plug isn't released, abort the mission. Using fingertips and a clean, dry cotton pad, gently press around clogged pores to remove surface debris.

- **Astringent:** Wipe the skin clean with a mild, alcohol-free toner to remove any residue.

- **Mask:** Apply a clay- or mud-based purifying mask. Leave on the face for ten minutes.

- **Spray:** Wipe off the mask with a warm washcloth and follow with a cooling mist to close pores.

Maintenance is important to keep skin clear. A combination of at-home and professional treatments works best.

TOP TIP:

Instead of frequent salon facials, switch to microdermabrasion (see page 56). Don't have a treatment when your skin flares up.

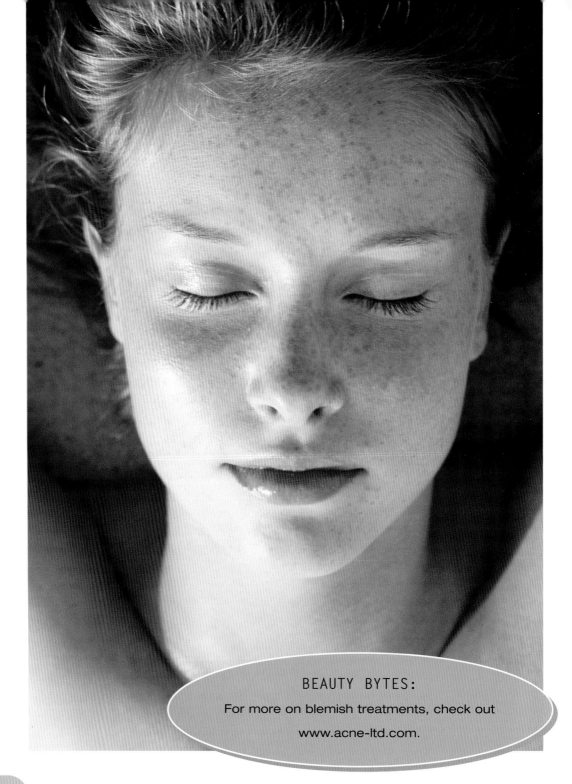

BEAUTY BYTES:

For more on blemish treatments, check out

www.acne-ltd.com.

back acne regime

What could be worse than blemishes on your back that show up just when you want to wear a skimpy top? If you're prone to "bacne," ask a friend to check out areas you can't get to on your own.

- **DO** pat dry. Don't wipe or rub vigorously, as this can irritate.

- **DO** wash twice daily with a BHA-based cleanser.

- **DO** wipe the affected area with a benzoyl peroxide or salicylic acid pad.

- **DO** follow with an AHA-based body lotion to help exfoliate skin while preventing it from drying out.

- **DO** use a salicylic acid or benzoyl peroxide skin treatment on individual areas at night.

- **DON'T** ever pick or squeeze pimples on the back or chest, where the skin is thicker and more prone to scarring.

- **DON'T** forget to shower as soon as possible after perspiring from sports, swimming, sunning, or other physical exertion.

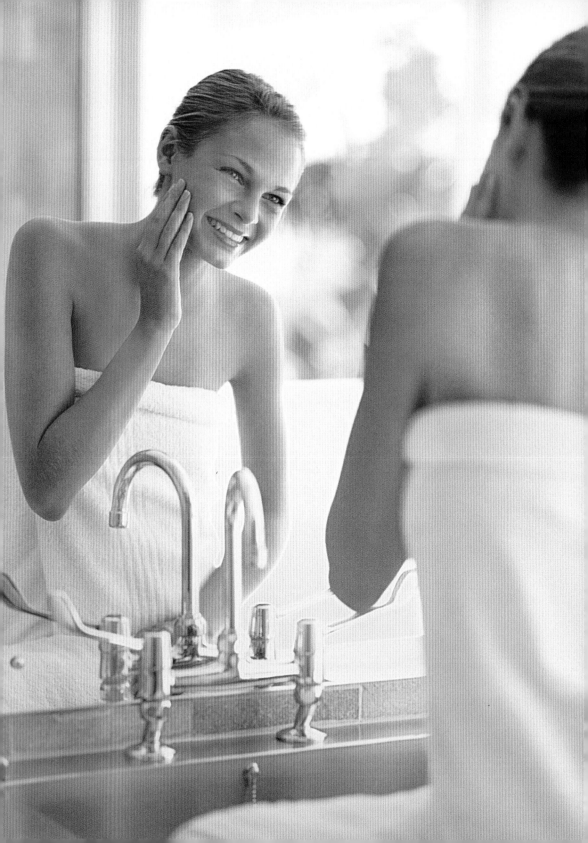

BANISHING BLEMISHES

No one has to suffer with acne. Help is available in many forms. Effective over-the-counter treatments have taken center stage. Finding a treatment best suited to your needs can take a lot of trial and error. Using too much or the wrong formula can give your face a shiny look and clog pores. Acne can't be cured completely, but it can be successfully controlled through consistent use of the right products.

Over-the-counter treatments for mild to moderate acne work by reducing the amount of oil produced and by reducing the bacteria that cause infection. Antibacterials prevent infection from spreading. Anti-inflammatories reduce swelling, redness, and inflammation. Keratolytics normalize the shedding of the follicle lining and remove dead cells. Of the nonprescription treatment options available, oil absorbers keep shine to a minimum and drying agents help reduce oil plugs and keep pores unclogged.

For acne sufferers who have dry or sensitive skin, even though they have pimples, any drying product may be too irritating.

drying out

Although there is a huge variety of acne treatments on the market, the majority contain various concentrations of the same vital ingredients.

Prescription and over-the-counter benzoyl peroxide treatments work in the same way, but prescription formulas often have higher concentrations. It is prescribed most often to make sure patients get the best formulation for their type of acne—in a cream, gel, or lotion. Benzoyl peroxide kills bacteria and reduces oil production. Salicylic acid, sulfur, and resourcinol help dissolve blackheads and whiteheads. Topical medicines, such as over-the-counter creams and gels, are applied directly onto the pimples or pimple-prone areas. Most of these help to dry out the excess oil and block the spread of infection. For mild acne, doctors often recommend using an over-the-counter remedy before resorting to more serious treatments that require a prescription. Be patient. It may take a month to see results from over-the-counter products.

Benzoyl peroxide
Concentration 2.5, 5, 10
Kills bacteria, removes shedding cells from follicle

Benzoyl peroxide destroys the *P. acnes* bacteria by penetrating the follicle and releasing hydrogen peroxide. For more than just a few blemishes, spread a thin film of cream or ointment over the entire area to prevent the acne from spreading. Benzoyl peroxide's main drawback is that it can cause irritation, dryness, peeling, or redness, and many women stop using it for that reason.

blushing beauty

Your face flushes unexpectedly, the broken blood vessels in your cheeks get red and swollen, you get flare-ups of bumps or pimples, and sometimes a stinging or burning.

These symptoms may last for hours or days and start up without warning. The bad news is that it sounds like rosacea, a chronic skin condition that has no cure. The good news is that rosacea can be treated, and should be. If left untreated, it will usually get worse. Rosacea is generally diagnosed by what stage it is in; first (mild), second (moderate) or third (severe). It starts later in life than acne and affects the cheeks, chin, nose, and forehead.

No cause has been definitively linked with rosacea, which makes it difficult to figure out. It is considered a vascular disorder and can be brought on by menopause, high blood pressure, stress, or fever. Like most other skin afflictions, it is more common in women than in men. At least 25 percent of women in their thirties and forties have rosacea. Statistics indicate that rosacea now ranks as the fifth most common diagnosis made by dermatologists, and it is still considered widely underdiagnosed.

People most prone to rosacea are aged between thirty and sixty, of Irish, English, or Scottish descent, or with northern or eastern European origins, fair skinned, with a family history of rosacea. Having had an adverse reaction to an acne medication or a sty may also be indications.

get the red out

Rosacea is basically a vascular problem, which is why you may appear red and flushed. Thin skin reveals the enlarged veins that lie underneath the surface.

Treatments for rosacea range from topical antibiotics to retinoids, peels, lasers, sclerotherapy injections, and light sources. Light glycolic acid peels are often used in conjunction with antibiotics to control rosacea. A series of peels are performed every two to four weeks along with a skin care program with washes and creams that have a low concentration of glycolic acid.

Tiny facial veins called "telangiectasias" can be effectively zapped with lasers that emit specific wavelengths of light that target the visible blood vessels just under the skin. Heat from the laser's energy builds in the vessels, causing them to collapse. More than one treatment may be needed, and with the most advanced lasers and laser light devices, there is little or no bruising. Once you've zapped the existing blood vessels, you will need additional treatments for new ones as they crop up.

Lasers also work for rhinophyma, a severe stage of rosacea that causes the tip of the nose to swell and the skin to become thickened and bulbous. Fortunately for women, this is much more common in men.

BEAUTY BYTES:

If you think you might have rosacea, check out www.rosacea.org.

operation avoidance

There is a definite distinction between rosacea and run-of-the-mill sensitive skin, although if you have rosacea, your skin might be sensitive and reactive.

Conquering rosacea usually means avoiding anything that may bring on an attack. Culprits vary from person to person. Wash thoroughly with a soap-free cleanser and lukewarm water to prevent fungal infections: Rosacea medications kill bacteria, creating new space for fungi to grow. Be sensible about what you put on your face in terms of skin care and makeup. Metronidazole (in the form of Metrogel or Noritate) is commonly prescribed, as are certain retinoids.

Things to avoid:

Lifestyle	Sun exposure (Public Enemy #1) • Cold and wind • Saunas, hot tubs, and steamy showers • Getting overheated • Coughing or straining • Loofahs, sponges, washcloths, and abrasives • Smoking
Skin care ingredients	Alcohol • Fragrance • Menthol • Witch hazel • Peppermint oil • Detergents • Acids • Chemical sunscreens • Astringents
Diet	Very hot caffeinated drinks (tea, coffee, hot chocolate) • Foods high in niacin (liver, yeast) • Foods containing histamines (tomatoes, eggplant, cheese) • Spices (paprika, chili, cayenne, Asian mustard) • Alcoholic beverages (wine, beer, liquor)

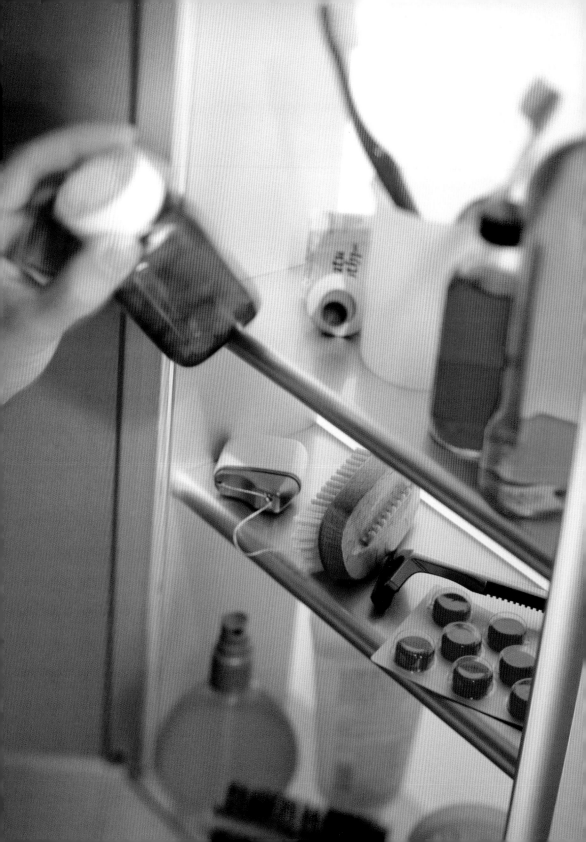

AT THE SKIN DOCTOR

When curing acne, there comes a time when only prescription medicines will do. With a dermatologist's help, most cases of acne can be cleared up, at least temporarily. Over-the-counter products may offer relief from some forms of acne, but won't clear up cysts lying deep within the skin or prevent new eruptions from appearing. If you have a chronic problem that won't go away on its own and doesn't respond to your regime, see a dermatologist. Don't let it get out of control. A doctor can treat your acne from the inside out with oral and topical medications. No one should have to suffer with acne indefinitely when there are safe and effective medications available.

Most prescription topical medications come in a variety of forms. Moisturizing creams and lotions are good for people with dry skin. Alcohol-based gels and solutions tend to be drying, so are best for oily skin. All forms work to reduce sebum production, ease inflammation, kill bacteria, and stabilize the androgen level. For eruptions in harder-to-reach areas like the back or shoulders, oral medication may be easier to use than topical antibiotics. Topical vitamin A derivatives are still considered the cornerstone of an anti-acne treatment plan among dermatologists.

in the clear

The biggest mistake women make is waiting it out. The earlier you seek treatment, the less chance of scarring. Antibiotics are the most common place to start.

Antibiotics are often used together with other therapies in a capsule form. They work to destroy *P. acnes* bacteria to reduce inflammation, redness, and pus formation. In many cases, you will need to stay on oral antibiotics for two to four months at a time. Always finish the prescription; if it is interrupted, it may become ineffective. You should follow the directions for taking your medication to the letter. Some antibiotics should be taken on an empty stomach; others are more effective when they are taken with or after meals. You might be told to take them at least one hour before bedtime. Your doctor may advise you not to take other medications or supplements—like iron or calcium—while taking some antibiotics, because they can interfere with absorption. Certain types, like the tetracyclines, are harder on the digestive tract, while others are more slowly absorbed and may have fewer side effects. If you are having trouble using the antibiotic prescribed, speak to your doctor about changing your medication. If your acne comes back while you are taking antibiotics that were previously helpful, you may have become resistant to them. Your doctor may want to switch you to a different class of antibiotics. Cream, lotion, and gel formulas are commonly used in addition to pills as antibacterial agents.

Side effects: Nausea or diarrhea, sun sensitivity, yeast infections, headache, dizziness, skin discoloration, tooth discoloration.

Oral antibiotics

Drug Class	Brand Name
Tetracycline	Tetracycline, Achromycin, Sumycin
Doxycycline	Doryx, Vibramycin
Minocycline	Dynacin, Minocin, Vectrin
Erythromycin	E-mycin, Ery-C, Ery-tab, E.E.S., Ery-ped, Erthrocin, PCE
Penicillin-type drugs	Ampicillin, Cephalexin
Sulfa	Bactrim, Cotrim, Septra

This is a partial list to be used as a guide. Not all drugs are available in all countries, and generic and brand names vary. Some medications that require a prescription in the United States are available over the counter in other countries. Check with your doctor or pharmacist to find out what medications are available to you.

Hormone therapy is used to reduce the amount of androgens in a woman's body, most commonly through birth control pills. Low-dose corticosteroid drugs, such as prednisone or dexamethasone, may have an anti-inflammatory effect and suppress the androgen produced by the adrenal glands. Antiandrogen medications, such as Spironolactone, may be prescribed to help prevent androgens from causing excessive oil production.

Side effects: Menstrual irregularities, breast tenderness, headache, fatigue.

the A list

Retinoids are derivatives of vitamin A that work to unclog pores. Retin-A has been on the market since the 1970s and is commonly used to treat wrinkles, psoriasis, and acne.

Retinoids treat blackheads and whiteheads effectively and fight acne by increasing cell turnover, which helps unplug existing comedos so that other topical medications, such as antibiotics, can penetrate the follicles better. In the United States, a prescription is required, but in some countries, prescription-strength retinoids are sold over the counter. One downside is that retinoids can dry out the skin and cause peeling and irritation. The acne can worsen during the first month of treatment because the medication draws out eruptions that would not otherwise have shown up yet. These side effects usually decrease or disappear when the medication has been used for a while and your skin is used to it. Many women worry that Retin-A will "thin the skin." Tretinoin causes a thinning of the epidermis, or outer layer of skin. It is an exfoliating agent or keratolytic, which makes it effective in removing the oil plugs that cause acne blemishes.

How to use retinoids:
Wait a half hour after cleansing to apply. Apply sparingly and at night. A pea-sized dab is enough for your entire face. Apply sunscreen before going out.

New kids on the block include Tazarotene (Tazorac), a potent synthetic retinoid, and Adapalene (Differin), a topical compound that helps decrease microcomedone formation.

Topical acne drugs

Types of drug	Brand Name	Form
Tazarotene	Tazorac	Cream, gel
Thromycin	ATS	Solution, gel
Erythromycin	Erycette	Pads
	Erygel	Gel
	Erymax	Solution
	Staticin	Solution
	T-Stat	Cream
Clindamycin Phosphate	Cleocin T	Solution, gel, pads
Sulfacetamide	Klaron	Lotion
Sulfur	Sulfacet-R	Lotion
Metronidazole	Metrogel	Gel, cream, lotion
Adapalene	Differin	Gel, pads, cream
Tretinoin	Retin-A	Cream, gel, lotion
	Retin-A Micro	Gel
	Avita	Cream, gel
Azelaic Acid	Azelex	Cream

This is a partial list to be used as a guide. Not all drugs are available in all countries and generic and brand names vary. Some medications that require a prescription in the United States are available over the counter in other countries. Check with your doctor or pharmacist to find out what medications are available to you.

the last resort

Isotretinoin is used as a last resort to clear up severe, cystic acne. Now available for over twenty years, Isotretinoin has been shown to be effective for 70–85 percent of patients.

Isotretinoin, or Accutane, is the closest thing we have to an acne cure. It comes in 10-, 20-, or 40-milligram capsules that are taken with food once or twice daily. The average treatment period is four months and the strength and frequency is determined by your doctor. Additional treatment courses can be given for recurrences. The most likely candidate for repeat treatments is suffering from deep, painful, cystic acne that has not responded to the usual alternatives.

When all else fails, many acne sufferers turn to Accutane to clear their complexions. It is currently the only medication that actually shrinks the gland that produces the oily sebum found in acne. Accutane is a potent drug that often produces dramatic results, but it also comes with some serious side effects and risks. Among the more serious of these are elevated blood cholesterol, lipid, and triglyceride levels, and abnormal liver enzymes. The side effects you may experience usually go away after the medication is stopped.

BEAUTY BYTES:

For information about Accutane, log on to

www.rocheusa.com.

Careful screening and evaluation will be done before you can start taking the drug, as well as close monitoring and frequent blood tests during therapy. If you have difficulty tolerating it, your doctor may be able to reduce the dose of the drug so that the side effects are reduced or stopped. You will be instructed not to take other vitamin A derivatives while you are using this medicine, including supplements containing beta-carotene.

If you are using ANY form of retinoid therapy, there is increased sensitivity to the sun because the epidermis is thinner. Sunscreen with a minimum SPF 15 is a must. Sun exposure can cause severe irritation or burning and lead to hyperpigmentation and possible scarring.

Side effects: Dry eyes, dry mouth, dry skin, cracked, peeling lips, itching, nosebleeds, muscle aches, depression.

Topical Accutane is being used in Canada and Europe, and may soon be available in the United States as well.

WARNING: Don't even think about getting pregnant while taking Accutane. This drug cannot be taken during pregnancy or while breast-feeding because it can cause severe birth defects.

peels with appeal

Chemical peels are used to unroof pustules and exfoliate the skin. Exfoliation helps topical treatments to penetrate the skin in order to control acne and prevent further outbreaks.

Peeling principles are based on the fact that the cells in the epidermis regenerate every month. Peels cause a burn in the skin similar to sunburn, depending upon the type of compound used and its concentration. The top layers of skin—epidermis and dermis—are scraped off. New skin cells begin to form a new top layer twenty-four hours after the procedure. One to two days later more new cells, called fibroblastic cells, become active in the dermis. These cells create new collagen fibers, which constitute the support structure of the newly generated skin. At the same time, the elastin fibers, which give the skin its flexibility, also begin to regenerate. Peels of sufficient depth can produce inflammation, redness of the skin, and swelling. Peeling agents that reach the deeper layers of the skin cause some degree of injury, and then actually peel off some of the cells in the epidermis.

Most superficial to moderate peels are performed in the doctor's office, and the procedure takes about thirty minutes. It begins with deep skin cleansing, after which the peeling compound is applied. This remains on the skin for a few minutes, causing burning and stinging. Light peels are typically repeated at intervals of three to four weeks, until the desired effect is achieved. A monthly or bimonthly maintenance program will help keep acne under control, and between-treatment creams that contain

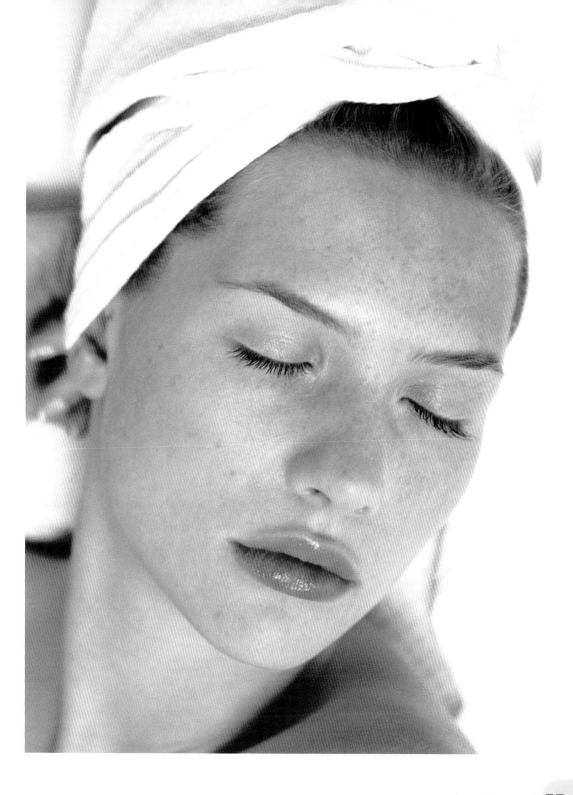

retinoic or glycolic acid should be used regularly to preserve the results of the treatment. One significant advantage of superficial peels over medium or deep peels is the lack of downtime. Superficial or "lunchtime" peeling revitalizes the outer layers of skin for a smooth, rejuvenated appearance. Medium-depth peeling is usually recommended for fair-skinned individuals, but superficial face peels can be done on all skin types. For acne, peeling can considerably reduce the number of blemishes and can improve skin color, transforming it from sallow and dull to radiant and smooth.

Alpha hydroxy acid (AHA): Superficial glycolic peels can be repeated as needed, to exfoliate and keep pores open and clean. Daily use of a peel with a glycolic acid–based lotion will contribute to continued clearing of the skin.

Beta hydroxy acid (BHA): Salicylic acid, the ingredient in aspirin, is often used to treat acne because it reduces inflammation as well as blackheads and pimples. Salicylic acid is oil soluble and can therefore penetrate oil-plugged pores.

Trichloracetic acid (TCA): A deep peel that penetrates into the dermis, TCA lightens pigmented acne scars and evens out skin tone. A TCA peel is usually done once every few months. Deep TCA peels produce burning, redness, and peeling that are more severe, and may take a week or more to heal.

Microdermabrasion: A state-of-the-art peel that uses a high-powered combination of force plus suction to deliver finely ground aluminum oxide or sodium crystals to give the skin a remarkably smooth texture. It can reduce acne and related scarring, enlarged pores, and surface lesions, and forestall eruptions.

let there be light

Moving beyond the pharmacy, light-based therapies may offer the next wave in skin-clearing treatments. The future looks bright.

New technologies emit a narrow band spectrum of intense violet-blue light to destroy bacteria found in acne. When the high-intensity lamp is shined directly on the skin, it kills the bacteria. These devices may be able to achieve better results than antibiotics and destroy acne-causing bacteria for a few months. Another system uses a green wavelength of heat and light over the face and body to clear acne by stimulating the body's natural defenses against acne by producing oxygen. Treatments are done twice a week for four weeks, followed by a maintenance program. Topical medications can be used in conjunction with light therapy when needed.

Laser treatments for acne that deliver energy down to the oil-producing centers in the sebaceous glands can destroy these oil reservoirs without causing heat damage that can harm the outer layers of the skin. They have the potential to offer a faster, more controlled treatment of severe acne and cystic acne, as an alternative to traditional topical or oral medicines without the side effects.

BEAUTY BYTES:

For more information about light therapy, log on to www.acneworld.com.

wrinkles and acne

As if puberty wasn't tough enough, what do you do when you can't decide whether wrinkles or blemishes are your biggest skin-care concern?

You've got crow's-feet and frown lines, as well as pimples on your cheeks, chin, and forehead. While the demand for antiwrinkle products increases steadily, women have an insatiable appetite for new and improved acne therapies.

Skin has a pH balance of 5.5. If you're mistreating your skin by using harsh detergents, overcleansing, overscrubbing, or layering on acids, your pH may climb to 7.5 or higher. Healthy skin will bounce back quickly, but if your skin is under siege, it can take longer to recover, leaving it more susceptible to stress. A normal pH of 5.5 protects skin from bacteria, which tend to thrive in a more alkaline environment. It is important to keep the skin moisturized while treating the eruptions. The areas of the face that contain the fewest oil glands, like around the eyes and the neck, need hydration. Use a noncomedogenic moisturizer for dry areas.

For mature skins suffering from lines and lesions, the name of the game is gentle exfoliation. In these cases, mild forms of vitamin A like a low dose of prescription-strength tretinoin or over-the-counter retinols are ideal. They can work within the skin's surface where wrinkles start. Combined with a gentle formula of AHAs and BHAs, you can keep pores clean and keep future eruptions at bay.

Regrettably, adult acne is more common in women than in men. If your adult acne breakouts are chronic or severe, do not delay seeing a dermatologist to design a prescription program that can effectively reduce oil production, fight bacterial infection, and jump-start your rate of cell renewal. Women over forty often respond well to oral antibiotics like tetracycline, doxycycline, or minocycline, as well as milder retinoids like Retin-A Micro and Avita.

The newer, kinder, gentler topical acne formulas are more cosmetically elegant, which makes them ideal for mature skin. They can be worn discreetly under foundation without some of the redness and irritation you may have experienced earlier. Cream formulas are used more frequently than gels, which are reserved for oilier skin types. If you were treated with Accutane in your teens and twenties, another course may be recommended to clear up your skin now.

If you get occasional eruptions but more often during warmer months or in humid weather, the first place to start is by adjusting your skin care routine. The challenge in treating wrinkle- and acne-prone skin is to control breakouts and keep pores clear and refined, while keeping skin hydrated and supple.

The first task at hand is to get the oil under control by gently targeting blemish-prone areas. Then keep drier, wrinkle-prone areas, like around the eyes, neck, and upper lip, well nourished by adding light moisturizing products that won't clog pores. Trade in heavy wrinkle creams for oil-free lotions, foundations, and sunscreens. Add a BHA-based gel or lotion, and use a tea tree oil or benzoyl peroxide spot treatment to dab on several times a day over or under makeup that can reduce redness and zap zits fast.

EXPERT ADVICE:

It's easy to think you have acne when it is another skin condition entirely. Perioral dermatitis can show up on the chin as little blisters.

skin care questions

skin care questions

Keep a journal of your acne history—what worked and what didn't, when your acne seems to flare up, and potential causes. A dermatologist will evaluate the severity of your acne and suggest the therapy that has had the most success in the treatment of cases similar to yours.

Questions you should ask your doctor:

- Are there better medications to clear up my acne than the ones I've tried?

- How long will it take for my acne to clear up?

- How often should I wash the affected area?

- What is the next step if this method doesn't work effectively?

- What is the best combination of medications for my type of acne?

- What cosmetic and skin care ingredients should I avoid?

- Should I avoid certain foods?

- What else can I do to help clear up my acne?

Questions your doctor might ask you:

- How long have you had acne?

- What skin products are you now using and have you used in the past?

- What medications are you currently taking?

- When do flare-ups most often occur?

- In what areas on your body and face do you have blemishes?

- Have you seen other doctors about it before?

- What treatments have you already tried?

- Did any of the treatments work? If so, which ones?

- Did your parents have acne when they were young?

- If so, how severe was their acne?

- Do you have a history of any hormonal imbalances?

- If so, what are your symptoms?

- How active are you and how much sun exposure do you get?

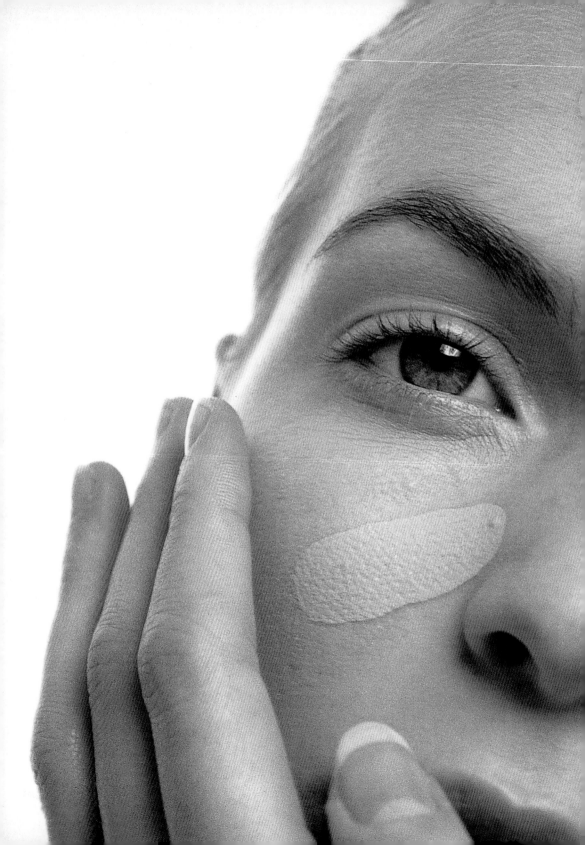

SCAR WARS

SCAR WARS

Old acne scars from your turbulent teens can ruin an otherwise smooth complexion at any age. The best way to prevent scars is to treat acne early, and for as long as is necessary. If left untreated, acne can cause significant scarring later on. Scars are the visible reminders of injury and tissue repair. In the case of acne, the injury is caused by the body's inflammatory response to sebum, bacteria, and dead cells in the plugged follicle.

Some people scar more easily than others and scarring varies from one person to the next. This marking of the skin frequently results from severe inflammatory cystic acne that occurs deep in the skin, and can also arise from more superficial pimples. Some women bear their acne scars for a lifetime and notice little change in them. In others, the skin undergoes some degree of remodeling and blemishes diminish in size. It is difficult to predict who will scar, how extensive or deep scars will be, how long they will persist, and how successfully scars can be prevented by effective treatment. The more inflammation can be prevented, the more likely it is that scarring can be avoided.

big squeeze

Keeping your hands off your face serves two purposes. It prevents the spread of bacteria that cause bad skin and helps you resist the temptation to squeeze, which causes scarring.

Squeezing forces infected material deeper into the skin, causing additional inflammation that takes longer to heal. Picking pimples will not help clear them up and may leave you with permanent scars. Tissue injured by squeezing can become infected by skin bacteria. Squeezing blackheads can also injure the sebaceous follicle and the tissue around it, and force it deeper as well as extruding it to the skin's surface. The result can be the start of an inflammatory reaction. Left on their own, blackheads do not usually get inflamed. Never squeeze your skin hard enough to leave an imprint.

Picking whiteheads is potentially even more harmful because they are more likely to become inflamed. Microcomedos are almost too small to be seen, but you can feel them as roughness on the skin. Once they become inflamed, they may develop into a pustule or a papule. Squeezing a microcomedo or closed comedo (whitehead) will not remove the contents anyway. A microcomedo is an undeveloped comedo, so there is really nothing there to squeeze out. A whitehead has such a small follicular opening that it is practically invisible, so little or no contents can be extruded. True cysts are nodules that rest deep below the skin's surface, so you can't get to them by squeezing your skin. Any attempt to manipulate them by prodding or picking will just aggravate the inflammatory process. If you've got cysts, the only effective therapy comes in a pill form.

saving face

One of the causes of scarring and delayed healing is skin fragility. Never squeeze your skin hard enough to leave an imprint.

When the melanocytes are disrupted, the skin needs outside help to come back to its normal state. Using your fingernails to pick can strip away pigmented cells from the deep layer of the skin and leave you with a very uneven skin tone in desperate need of blending and bleaching. Be careful about manipulating or picking away at areas of skin that are most prone to scarring, like the chin, chest, and back.

Don't apply concealer on blemishes or incisions that are open. They need to heal before you can cover up any remaining dark areas. If you have an open pimple, apply an acne-drying gel or lotion and let it run its course.

If you have uneven skin pigmentation, you need a product that contains at least 4 percent hydroquinone to be effective. Prescription hydroquinone inhibits the production of excessive pigment that can lead to dark spots. Other key bleaching agents include kojic acid, arbutin, licorice extract, L-ascorbic acid, tretinoin, glycolic acid, and azelaic acid. Irritation may occur from any of these. Lightening takes four to six weeks of continuous use to see improvement, and it may take three to four months for deeper areas of discoloration. Sun avoidance is key.

under cover

Cosmetic acne is less of a problem today because of the array of noncomedogenic products on the market. The right foundation and powder can actually absorb excess oil.

Oil-free foundations and concealers are a must. They can help cover up swelling and red blemishes as they heal, and actually speed up the process. It is often difficult to apply foundation during the first few weeks of treatment when skin is red or scaly from the remedies. Waterproof formulas don't come off with soap and water, and require more cleansing and rubbing to remove. These are not usually recommended for acne-prone skin. The trick is to NEVER go to bed without removing your makeup completely, so there is no residue left on the skin overnight.

Acne scars present a marathon challenge for makeup gurus trying to cover them effectively because they are generally not flat, but either raised or sunken. Carefully placed concealer with the right primer and foundation are essential for cheeks, chins, foreheads, and necks.

For depressed scars: Start with a primer to allow foundation to flow on smoothly. Applied with a sponge, foundation gives a flawless finish for recessed areas.

MAKEUP MUST-HAVE:

Powder compact and blotting papers for emergency oil spills.

For darkened or red scars: Start with a pale concealer, and add a second coat a few shades lighter than your skin. End with concealer that matches your skin, setting each layer with pressed powder.

makeup maneuvers

- Apply makeup to a face that has been cleansed and is completely dry.

- Only use oil-free foundation. On mature or combination skin, you can try a formula with a little oil. Use a small amount applied in five dots. One on the forehead, one on the tip of the nose, one on each cheek, and one on the chin.

- Gently pat dots of concealer that matches your skin tone under the eyes, on the lids, on any broken capillaries, or on very red, blemished areas. Use a camouflage brush or a cotton swab to blend it in. Green-tinted concealer can help to get the red out. Yellow is preferred for correcting bluish skin discolorations, dark circles under the eyes, and pasty complexions.

- Use a fine, matte powder all over the face, lids, and around the lips to control oil. Choose a shade that won't change the hue of your concealer. Even if you don't use foundation, powder is key.

- If you forget or skip the powder phase, the foundation will mix with the natural oils in your skin and melt. Foundation contains pigment particles that are broken down during the day.

scar remedies

Total restoration of the skin to the way it looked before acne first attacked is not always possible, but the skin surface can be improved to some extent.

The most common souvenir is uneven skin texture, especially visible on the soft areas of the face like the cheeks. This is caused by tough scar tissue that forms both on the surface and in the deep skin layers. Acne erupts from the deep tissue to the surface of the skin, so the scars left behind are more complex than those from cuts and scrapes. Acne scars are three-dimensional because they go through the skin. For depressed scars, fillers can be injected under the skin to elevate the scar and fill it in.

One of the causes of scarring and delayed healing is skin fragility. Using your fingernails to pick can strip

Acne scar fillers

Form	Brand Name
Human fat	
Human tissue	Cymetra, Fascian Cosmoplast
Bovine collagen	Zyplast, Zyderm
Bovine collagen with microparticles	ArteColl
Injectable liquid silicone	Silskin Silikon 1000
Hyaluronic acid	Restylane Perlane Hylaform Hylaform Plus

away pigmented cells from the deep layer of the skin and leave you with a very uneven skin tone in desperate need of blending and bleaching.

Dark skin types are even more susceptible to "postinflammatory hyper-pigmentation"—doc-speak for dark blotches that often show up on darker skin types after acne lesions heal, and seem to take forever to clear, if at all. When melanocytes, which form the original color of the skin, are disrupted, the skin needs outside help to return to its normal state, in the form of exfoliating and bleaching agents, to effectively lighten darkened areas so they blend in with the rest of your complexion. Total sun protection is a must for dark spots, as sun exposure will turn them darker and make them last longer.

The darker your skin, the darker the hyperpigmentation is likely to be and the longer it will take to lighten. Bleaching dark spots takes months, so be patient. Black skin is prone to scarring and dark blotches. It discolors quickly. Asian skin has yellow undertones and is transparent and soft, so it magnifies every mark. Latin skin is firm, tough, and generally oilier.

Many of the treatments used to keep acne under control are also helpful in taking care of the scars it leaves behind, only in a deeper mode.

Microdermabrasion uses aluminum oxide crystals passing through a vacuum tube to remove surface skin and smooth down ridges. Multiple procedures, often deeper than the customary treatments, will be needed to soften acne scarring.

Dermabrasion involves using a high-speed brush to remove surface skin and alter the contour of deep scars. In dark-skinned people, dermabrasion may cause changes in pigmentation that require additional treatment. It is less common today due to the advent of lasers.

Chemical peels in a series of glycolic acid, beta hydroxy acid, and trichloracetic acid (TCA) can be used in varying strengths to improve the appearance of scars left from acne lesions.

Ablative lasers

Lasers of various wavelengths and intensities are used to recontour scar tissue and reduce the redness around healed acne lesions. Ablative laser technologies can improve the deepest scars that remain decades after acne has run its course. In some cases, a single treatment will achieve permanent results. The downside is that because the skin absorbs bursts of energy from the laser, there may be redness for several months. The CO_2 laser vaporizes thin layers of the skin and tightens collagen fibers, which is good for depressed acne scars. The Erbium:YAG laser produces very precise bursts of energy, which allows for the sculpting of smaller, irregular scars. CO_2 laser–treated sites heal in seven to ten days, while skin treated with the Erbium:YAG laser heals in five to seven days. Coblation, which uses low-energy frequency to treat scars, falls somewhere between CO_2 and Erbium lasers. It can be used to produce some results on deep scars with less of a healing period than CO_2.

Nonablative lasers

Nonablative lasers are showing promise in softening acne scars, but they work slower. The cooling infrared lasers like CoolTouch cause mild redness for a few hours after the procedure, but no pain. The treatment feels like a rubber band lightly snapping against the skin with an alternating cool and warm sensation. An average of four treatments is required to reduce most acne scars, and they should be continued monthly as needed. The laser stimulates the body to produce more collagen under the skin. The deeper the scar, the more collagen you have to make to raise the scar up. Less intense lasers don't give immediate results because the collagen takes months to tighten. Intense Pulsed Light sources and Pulse Dye lasers offer quick treatment alternatives without the downtime, but they must be done in a series to improve scarring. For scars that have turned white over time, the Excimer laser has proved effective in repigmenting scar tissue, which is particularly useful for dark skin types more prone to hypopigmentation (skin lightening). Combination therapy with a series of laser or light-based treatments and mechanical resurfacing like microdermabrasion can be effective on large, soft areas of the face with rolling scar tissue. The light from a subsurfacing laser is used to stimulate new collagen growth in the deep layers of the skin, which can plump out any depressions left from scars.

Skin surgery

Some individual scars may be removed by a punch excision. The scar is excised down to the layer of fat underneath the skin; the resulting hole in the skin may be repaired with sutures or with a small skin graft. "Subcision" is a technique in which a surgical probe is used to lift the scar tissue away from unscarred skin, to elevate the depressed scar.

In older women with a history of acne and acne scarring, sometimes a face-lift will be recommended to stretch out the skin, which can soften some of the scars. Fillers like fat can be added to smooth out the deepest scars at the same time.

TOP TIP:
The best remedy for acne scars is a series of treatments or a combination of several therapies.

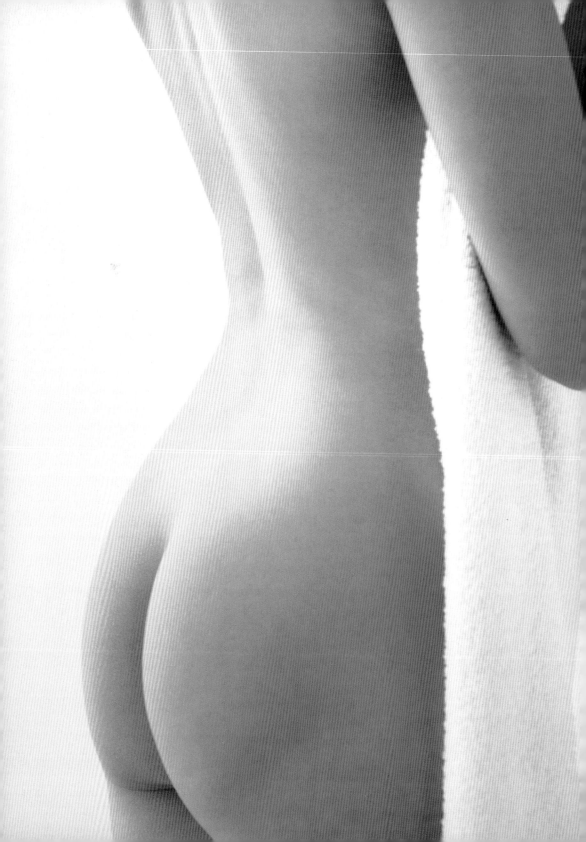

FIGURE IT OUT

FIGURE IT OUT

For centuries, women have been at war with their fat cells. Doctors estimate that more than half of us are heavier than we should be, and about one quarter are obese. Clearly, we're eating too much and moving too little. Many of us sit in front of computers all day, then go home and surf the Internet some more or sit in front of the TV until bedtime. In spite of the constant bombardment of signals to eat less food and more healthily and to exercise, many women are gaining weight faster and are getting heavier by the day. Studies show that being overweight increases your risk of dying young by at least 50 percent, and you are more likely to have high blood pressure, high cholesterol, diabetes, asthma, arthritis, and some cancers, including breast and colon cancer.

Losing weight isn't that hard; the difficult part is keeping it off. All too often, our idea of a shape-up program consists of jumping on the latest fad diet bandwagon, which we inevitably fall off when we get bored with it or it stops working. Plan on losing weight slowly and forget about looking for quick fixes. The ultimate measure of your success is your body fat percentage.

fat stats

Women have a basic love/hate relationship with fat. We are about 12 percent more likely to be obese than men and almost all of us are desperate to avoid becoming fat.

This sentiment accounts for the proliferation of diets, miracle pills, power drinks, and gym memberships. This three-letter word alone is enough to instill fear in the hearts of every woman with visions of lumps, bumps, bulges, and saddlebags. At any given time, between 15 and 35 percent of adults are dieting. Ninety percent of people with eating disorders are adolescents and young women. Fashion models weigh about one quarter less than the average female. We live in a culture in which fatness is considered tantamount to failure, and the pressure to be thin is very real to most women. Size still matters when it comes to determining self-worth or attractiveness. A woman's dress size has become inextricably linked with her identity. There are some women who don't store fat and can consume twice as many calories as the rest of us without gaining an ounce. No one said life is fair. The good news is that many women aren't as fat as they think they are.

Women struggle to control their fat, and will go to great lengths to lose it to the point of starvation. Everyone knows that the safest way to lose weight is to eat a nutritionally complete diet, low in calories and fat. Burning off more calories than you take in will cause you to lose weight. If you lose the weight slowly, you'll be much more effective at keeping it off, especially if you incorporate exercise into your routine. Excess fat can be reduced by limiting caloric intake to a level below the energy exerted, or increasing physical activity. The bad news is that there is no magic formula, and there is no one diet or plan that works for everyone. The typical unhealthy diet is loaded with sugar and fats, but contains less than the recommended amounts of fruits and vegetables. Every diet seems to have one common underlying theme—french fries and chocolate cake are out.

Generally, an older body is a fatter body. An average twenty-year-old woman's body is 16.5 percent muscle, 47 percent nonmuscle lean tissue, 10 percent bone, and 26.5 percent fat. By comparison, the average twenty-something guy has 30 percent muscle and only 18 percent fat. The differences between women and men increase with age. Both sexes become fatter, but women become more so. Excess fat settles in different places at different stages of life. The major culprit is estrogen.

Teens and 20s: Any excess fat is distributed evenly around your body.
30s and 40s: Extra weight goes straight to your hips and thighs.
50s: Added pounds head for your waistline and stay put.
60s and 70s: If you have been steadily gaining weight through the years, expect to be somewhat pear-shaped.

The older you get, the harder it is to lose weight because your body settles in, gets lazy, and grows accustomed to your fat. The shifting also tends to follow the pattern of gravity—it gets lower. In general, there is a tendency for the shoulders to narrow, the chest size to grow, and the pelvis to widen over the years. Chest size in women peaks between the ages of fifty-five and sixty-four. Although a bigger chest may seem like something to look forward to, it is usually accompanied by the flattening and sagging of the breasts. After age sixty-five, a woman's chest generally shrinks. The pelvis, in contrast, keeps widening throughout life, which accounts for the pear-shape period.

body mass

Body weight represents a sum of the bodily structures including muscle, bone, body water, and stored fat. One measure of plumpness is the dreaded Body Mass Index (BMI), which, at first glance, reads like an Einstein theory in physics.

BMI is determined by dividing weight in pounds by height in inches squared, then multiplying by 705. For example, a woman who is 5 feet 6 inches tall and weighs 189 pounds would have a BMI of 30.6. You are considered overweight if your BMI is 25–29.9, obese if you have a BMI of 30 or higher. However, not every woman fits neatly into BMI charts or height/weight statistics. If you have a large amount of muscle, which weighs more than fat, for example, your weight may seem higher than normal limits.

Lean body mass is commonly used to describe the muscles in your arms, legs, back, neck, and abdomen. Another measure doctors use is your body composition, which is your proportion of fat to muscle. A woman needs to have a minimum of 13–17 percent body fat for regular menstruation. If it is lower than that, periods may stop and you could become infertile. Menstrual cycle irregularities may also compromise healthy bones. The healthy ranges of body fat are significantly higher for women than for men, and the range increases slightly with age. For women, if your body fat is greater than 27–30 percent, you would be considered overweight.

BODY MASS INDEX

5 ft. 6 in. = 66 in.

66 in. x 66 in. = 4,356 sq. in.

189 pounds ÷ 4,356 = .0434

.0434 x 705 = 30.6 BMI

Not all fat is created equal

We all need some fat. It is vital for the maintenance of healthy skin and hair. Although everyone has a smooth layer of fat, individual amounts depend on weight, lifestyle, and genetics. This fat layer is an insulator for the body and cushions the organs,

Age	Healthy range of body fat
18–39	21–32%
40–59	23–33%
60–79	24–35%

muscles, and nerves to protect them from injury. Cellulite, on the other hand, is lumpy and provides no padding whatsoever. Then there is the visceral fat that can collect around the midsection and surround the organs. This can present the greatest risk to your health. Lipids seep into the bloodstream from this layer and can cause high cholesterol and cardiovascular disease.

Essential fat is found in small amounts in your bone marrow, organs, central nervous system, and muscles.

Storage fat is fat accumulated primarily beneath the skin but is also found in other areas in the body.

"False fat," the bloating that comes from hypersensitivity to many common foods, can create excess weight. We feel and look a lot better without it. It also comes off fastest. The loss of false fat is one of the reasons people sometimes lose weight quickly at the beginning of a new diet.

In 1996, Olestra, made with soybean or cottonseed oil, was approved by the FDA for use in snacks. Its chemical composition adds no fat or calories. A one-ounce serving of potato chips fried with Olestra contains seventy-five calories and no fat, as opposed to the normal 150 calories and ten grams of fat. Olestra may cause abdominal cramping, loose stools, and inhibit the absorption of some nutrients like vitamins A, D, E, and K.

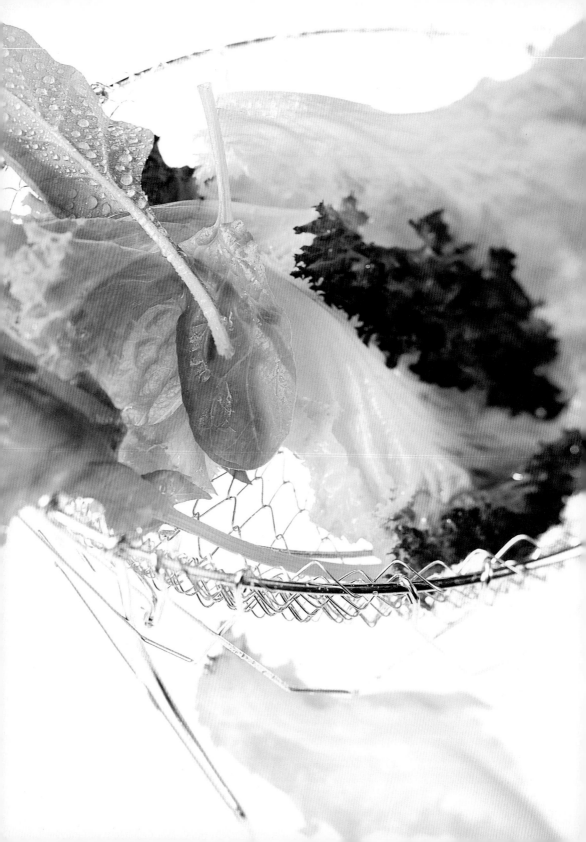

FAT FREEDOM

FAT FREEDOM

Fats are organic compounds made up of carbon, hydrogen, and oxygen, which belong to a group of substances called lipids. Fat provides nine calories per gram, more than twice the number provided by carbohydrates or protein. Fats provide the essential fatty acids, which are not made by the body and must be obtained from food. Fatty acids provide the raw materials that help in the control of blood pressure, blood clotting, inflammation, and other bodily functions, and are the primary components of dietary fats. Omega-3 fatty acid, or fish oil, is a polyunsaturated fat found in seafood, particularly fatty fish like salmon. This is a type of fat that helps increase healthy cholesterol, decrease bad cholesterol in the blood, and may lower blood pressure by lowering triglycerides.

Fat helps in the absorption of the fat-soluble vitamins A, D, and E, and helps maintain the immune system. You don't want to eliminate it completely, just limit what you take in to what you need and nothing more. The key is to strike a healthy balance. Success with your fat-loss mission depends primarily on nutrition, which is the first place to start. Next on the list is exercise.

never say diet

never say diet

In the last twenty years, the number of overweight women in their twenties has risen over 60 percent, and about half of all women in their thirties and forties are overweight.

Few of us live our lives at our ideal weight on a daily basis. Diets offer only short-term solutions; they are destined to become something you go on and come off because they are so limiting. The goal is to encourage long-term lifestyle changes.

It is difficult to maintain dramatic, significant weight loss for long periods. Set realistic goals. Aim for something that you feel can be maintained for six months. If you overindulge one day, don't waste precious time and energy feeling guilty, but get back on track the next day. If you're not sure you're really hungry, wait twenty minutes before you eat and you may find you weren't that hungry at all. Never let yourself get too famished or you'll be tempted to eat whatever is within reach.

Losing even as little as 5 to 10 percent of your body weight can make major health improvements. It helps glucose tolerance, blood pressure, and blood lipids because they improve on a continuum of weight loss. The simplest method is to decrease intake by 250 calories a day and increase expenditure by the same amount. If you exercise following weight loss, you will be more successful in keeping the weight off. Exercise changes the body so that it can handle fat, by burning it as a primary fuel. It also revs up your metabolism and turns your body into a fat-burning machine.

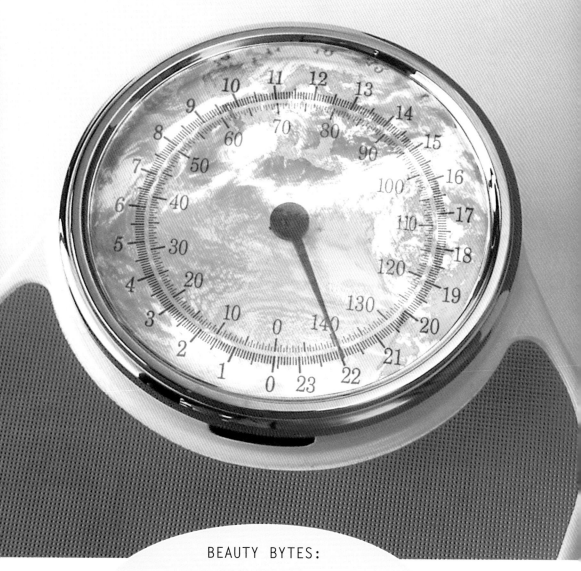

BEAUTY BYTES:

Need help planning a diet you can stick to?

Who doesn't? Log on to these sites:

www.ediets.com, www.cyberdiet.com,

www.nutrition.gov, and

www.ozgarcia.com.

just the fat

Counting fat grams is one way to get a clear picture of your daily totals. The trick is to maintain a diet of less than 30 percent fat.

"I'm eating fat-free foods, so why aren't I losing weight?" If that sounds familiar, you're not alone. Don't assume that because a food is called fat-free, you can eat as much as you want. Calories count, too. Nutritionists recommend reading labels and sticking to foods that have less than five fat grams. This allows you a treat of a few high-fat foods as long as they fit within your daily limit. If you only eat foods that are 30 percent fat or lower, your diet is guaranteed to be less than 30 percent fat, but that can be limiting. There will be times when you have a craving for something that measures higher than 30 percent.

Diets with less than 20 percent fat leave you unsatisfied and likely to overeat when willpower crumbles. Fat stimulates the release of a hormone that slows the rate of food leaving the stomach. The stomach is lined with receptors that signal the brain you're full when stimulated by fat. Fatty foods can be squeezed into a healthy diet if you only eat them in moderation as part of an otherwise low-fat diet. You can nibble a couple of cookies and still be OK, as long as you're not downing a pint of ice cream.

EXAMPLE

Total calories for day: 1950

Total fat grams: 36

36 fat grams x 9 calories per fat gram =
324 fat calories

Fat calories (324) ÷ total calories (2069) =
16.6% of total calories are
from fat

food diary

Sometimes putting it all on paper makes it official. At the end of the day, add up the fat grams and total calories. Work out your daily percentage by multiplying the fat grams by nine to get fat calories. Divide this number by the total calories. The final number should be less than 30 percent.

Day	Breakfast	Lunch	Dinner	Snacks	Calories	Fats
Monday						
Tuesday						
Wednesday						
Thursday						
Friday						
Saturday						
Sunday						

fat busters

Given the advances in "low-fat" and "nonfat" foods, it seems only fair that our waists should be shrinking.

It is common to think that if food is low in fat, you can eat twice as much or as much as you want. Sadly, this is not the case. Stick to "low-fat" and "fat-free" products whenever possible, and be skeptical about labels and claims. Note the serving size used when looking at nutritional information on packets. If the serving size is three ounces and you consume six ounces, remember to double the amount of fat, sugar, etc.

REALITY CHECK:
Alcohol can make you feel bloated and add on pounds. For example, a six-ounce glass of chardonnay contains 90 calories while eight ounces of beer has 150 calories.

Losing extra pounds involves more than counting calories and cutting back on fat. It's the little choices you make throughout the day that make or break your success. When it comes to weight loss, the number of calories count, no matter what the source. The bottom line is: Cut calories, increase exercise, lose weight. Many women spend most of their lives on yo-yo diets; the endless cycle of losing weight and gaining it back again. If you don't add resistance exercises to your program, you are going to lose muscle mass and will not get the results you desire.

Reading matters

What it says	What it means
Reduced fat	25% less fat than whatever it is being compared to
Light or lite	50% less fat than whatever it is being compared to
Low-fat	One serving has fewer than 3 grams of fat
Fat-free	One serving has less than 1/2 gram of fat
Lean (meats, seafood, poultry)	Less than 10 grams of fat, 4.5 grams of saturated fat, and 95 milligrams of cholesterol per serving and per 100 grams
Extra lean	Less than 5 grams of fat, 2 grams of saturated fat, and 95 milligrams of cholesterol per serving and 100 grams
Cholesterol-free	Less than 2 milligrams cholesterol and 2 grams or less saturated fat per serving
Low cholesterol	20 milligrams or less cholesterol per serving and 2 grams or less saturated fat per serving
High fiber	5 grams or more fiber per serving
Sugar-free	Less than 0.5 grams of sugar per serving
Sodium-free	Less than 5 milligrams sodium per serving
Low sodium	140 milligrams or less per serving
Light (in sodium)	50% reduction in sodium

magic bullets

Diet supplements, fat burners, and miracle pills come and go. Their mission is always the same: a cure for fat without any effort.

Drugs can produce weight loss for a while, but as soon as you stop taking them, the weight piles back on unless you have changed your ways. Pills can't change the way your body handles fat, they only make temporary adjustments.

Appetite suppressants

The medications most often used in the management of obesity are "appetite suppressants." These medications promote weight loss by decreasing appetite or increasing the feeling of being full. They decrease appetite by increasing serotonin or catecholamine, two brain chemicals that affect mood and appetite. Some antidepressants have also been used to this effect. Generally, these medications can lead to an average weight loss of 10–15 pounds above what would be expected by dieting alone. They are not recommended for someone who is mildly overweight or has less than 10 pounds to lose.

Every woman responds differently to appetite suppressants, and some experience more weight loss than others. Maximum weight loss usually occurs within the first six months, and then the weight loss tends to level off. Most appetite suppressants are recommended only for short-term use—a few weeks to a few months—and not for more than one year continuously. Sibutramine (Meridia) has been banned in some countries due to the risk factors effecting high blood pressure.

If you're considering appetite suppressant medication treatment, find out about potential risks. None of these medications come without their own set of side effects like irritability, sleeplessness, nervousness, dizziness, and elevations in blood pressure and pulse. Sometimes it is recommended to take the last dose during the afternoon to avoid trouble sleeping at night.

All prescription diet medications are "controlled substances," meaning doctors need to follow certain restrictions when prescribing them. Diet drugs are not magic bullets or a one-shot fix. They won't take the place of normal dieting and exercise. Their major role is to help you start and stay on a diet and exercise plan, to lose weight and keep it off. Many studies have also shown that the majority of people who stop taking appetite suppressant medications regain the weight they had lost. Medications should be taken only under strict medical supervision, and at the dosage directed. Buying them online and self-treating can be risky.

Fat blockers

Fat blockers are antiobesity drugs with the ability to stop foods from turning into fat cells within the body. This class of drugs is called "lipase inhibitors." They differ from other weight-loss drugs in that they block the breakdown and absorption of fat from the gastrointestinal tract. Because they allow fat to be excreted in the stool, there are possible side effects, such as bloating, diarrhea, and flatulence.

Orlistat (Xenical) is taken three times a day. Patients taking them are advised to take a supplement rich in the fat-soluble vitamins A, D, E, and K, and to curtail their fat intake. While taking these drugs, if you eat high-fat foods, the side effects increase. If you eat a meal that contains no fat or skip a meal, a dose of medication may be skipped.

get thin quick

If it sounds too good to be true, it is, especially when it comes to diets in a pill. Supplements alone will never get you svelte. You have to do your part.

We've all read the tempting claims; tablets that burn fat before food is digested, pills that help you lose two dress sizes without dieting or exercise, and products that burn body fat while you sleep. The list of "natural" diet aids includes vitamins, minerals, herbs, botanicals, teas, and other plant-derived substances, amino acids and concentrates, metabolites, constituents, and extracts of these substances. Their general mode of action is to burn fat by increasing the basal metabolic rate, which translates to burning more calories. Other products work by enhancing your energy levels, assisting with digestion, reducing your appetite, and easing water retention.

Nutritional supplements are not required to undergo the rigorous testing that a drug is subjected to, so manufacturers do not have to demonstrate that their product is either safe or effective. As a result, little is known about potential drug interactions, dosages, and long-term effects. Some of these potent ingredients can overtax your heart, increase your blood pressure, interfere with the heart's normal rhythm, or cause

BEAUTY BYTES:

To look up weight control supplements, log on to www.ephedra.com and www.webrx.com.

strokes. Other side effects include nervousness, anxiety, and insomnia. Among the most popular fat-loss formulas, ephedrine- and caffeine-based supplements have been linked with heart attacks and strokes, and kava kava has been cited as causing liver damage.

Supplements are products taken by mouth that contain a "dietary ingredient," which may include vitamins, minerals, herbs or other botanicals, amino acids, enzymes, metabolites, extracts, or concentrates, in many forms such as tablets, capsules, soft gels, gelcaps, liquids, powders, or bars. Manufacturers may make three types of claims: health, structure or function, and nutritional content. However, there are no regulations limiting serving size or the quantity of any nutrient.

The term "natural" does not guarantee that any product is safe. Look for ingredients in products with the U.S.P. notation, which indicates the manufacturer followed United States Pharmacopoeia guidelines. Consider the name of the manufacturer or distributor; supplements made by a nationally known food and drug manufacturer are more likely to be safe.

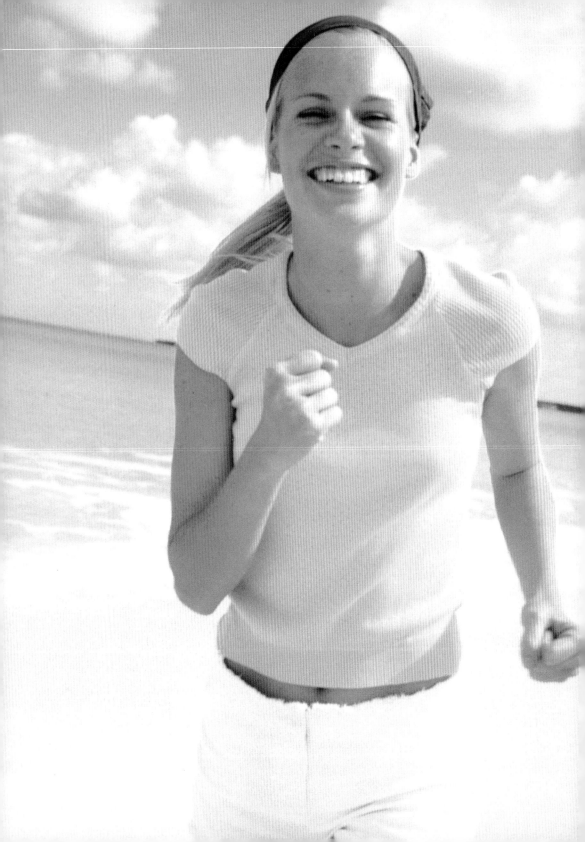

GET MOVING

GET MOVING

It should come as no surprise that from your twenties, muscle mass and metabolism decline. You can't eat the same way in your forties as you did in your twenties and expect to stay trim. Activity levels also tend to decrease with age. If you have a slow metabolism to start with, it becomes much harder to maintain your size as you get older. Add a couple of pregnancies and hormonal changes, and it takes a concentrated effort to avoid piling on the pounds. As you age, you have to be more careful about what you eat and increase your activity levels.

Even if you've never been to a gym, there is a workout that can keep you trim. If you've been inactive for a while, don't despair. Your muscles won't go to mush overnight. If you skip a week of exercise, you won't see much of a difference in your overall ability or strength. If you miss a month, you can expect to huff and puff a little more when you restart. If you skip three or four months, your body may need some retraining. Take it slowly—your aerobic strength and capability will have dropped a bit. If you've taken six months off, you'll be in the same cardiovascular shape as you were before you started exercising for the first time.

Women increase muscle mass with weight training, but not as much as men. Weight training causes favorable changes in body composition: better muscle tone and less fat. Your measurements confirm whether you're losing. The scale can't tell you how much is muscle or fat, and muscle weighs more.

keeping it off

Exercise is the most effective treatment for fat reduction. Committing to a regular exercise program also gives you the best chance of losing weight and keeping it off.

Many women look at their overweight parents and come to the conclusion: "I'm destined to be overweight and there's nothing I can do about it." Some of us have genes that predispose us to being overweight, and some overweight people may have an impaired metabolism that makes it harder, but neither of these facts preclude you from maintaining or losing weight.

Women who succeed in losing weight incorporate behavioral strategies into their regime: learning about nutrition, planning what to eat and when, and eating regular meals even between meetings and daily scheduling chaos. Exercise boosts weight loss because it builds muscle. Muscle tissue is the most metabolically active tissue in the body, so people with more muscles burn more calories, even when resting. It also increases your metabolic rate and keeps

TOP TIP:
Don't weigh yourself every day. Muscle is heavier than fat, so you won't see much change. Looking in the mirror and feeling your clothes getting looser is far more encouraging than the little number that registers on your bathroom scale. The best reward for losing a bit is treating yourself to a new outfit in a smaller size.

it elevated for a period even after you have finished working out. Beyond boosting caloric expenditure and moderating your appetite, exercise supports weight loss in other ways. It lowers your blood pressure, decreases your risk of diabetes, and improves your cardiovascular system. It also serves to keep your self-esteem high and your spirits up, and improves your overall body image. This sense of control contributes to reducing stress, which can trigger binge eating.

Exercise not only burns calories, but also improves glucose tolerance, which in turn moderates appetite. Glucose tolerance declines with excessive weight gain, making an extra carbohydrate load particularly destructive and increasing the likelihood of diabetes. Metabolic rate tends to decline after weight loss; when a large chunk of weight is lost quickly, more lean tissue is lost, which lowers your metabolic rate.

Use it to lose it

Take advantage of every opportunity to be active; take the steps instead of the elevator, walk instead of hailing a taxi, walk briskly instead of strolling, or park at the far end of the parking lot so you'll have to walk an extra sixty feet. Try to find some extra time in your day to sneak in a fifteen-minute jog or a quick aerobics class. Keep workout clothes in your office or car just in case the opportunity arises. At the end of the day, it all adds up.

Both weight training and cardiovascular exercise are essential. The more lean muscle tissue you have, the higher your resting metabolic rate will be. In other words, by developing more muscle, you will be burning more body fat all day long, even when you're not working out.

the bounce factor

Women have a smaller supply of the hormones that cause muscles to grow and develop, which is why men generally tend to be taller and more muscular.

Since women have more body fat, they typically have more fuel to burn off in endurance activities like running, cycling, swimming, and hiking. Ideally, combine aerobic activity that increases the heart rate with a resistance workout and weight training. Resistance exercise is good for muscle building, whereas aerobic exercise is better for reducing fat mass. Abdominal fat is most responsive to aerobics. Muscle fibers grow in response to the amount of work you make them do. If you're just starting to work with weights, anything you do will increase the amount of muscle you have on your frame. For example, you can do many repetitions at low resistance or fewer repetitions with more weight. As you get stronger, you can advance to the next level of resistance.

When it comes to burning off calories, people who do the same activity at the same pace for an equal amount of time can burn vastly different numbers of calories depending on their size. Generally, the larger you are, the more calories you burn, particularly from activities like walking or stair climbing, where you have to carry your own weight. Fat oxidation works best if your activity level is continuous. Exercise should ideally be low impact, at about 50–70 percent of cardiovascular endurance; for example, you should be breathless but still be able to talk while exercising.

lean on me

Resistance training builds up muscle and makes us stronger. Aerobic exercise stimulates the heart and increases the pulse rate. You need a little of both to get a good workout.

When you start any new form of training, your body will improve. But if you carry on working out in exactly the same way, using the same exercises, your body will adapt and stop improving at the same rate. Changing your workout routine will also keep it interesting. No matter what routine you follow, try to vary the intensity and duration of your workouts and the type of activities you do to get consistently good results. Using good technique will also ensure the best results from your program. Not doing your exercises in the right way won't help. Learn a few different ways to exercise each muscle group in case you can't get to the machine you want to use at the gym. To keep your workout effective and efficient, choose exercises that simultaneously work several major muscle groups. Your equipment should be easily accessible. Working out becomes a chore if you have to drive far to the gym.

REALITY CHECK:
Pick a starting point and aim for thirty minutes a day, five days a week—the minimum recommended by medical experts. You can begin with three days a week at low intensities and work your way up gradually. Ideally, exercise should be done seven days a week. Doing something as simple as walking for thirty minutes every day will help control your body weight.

tipping the scales

Exercise improves glucose tolerance, which in turn moderates appetite. Glucose tolerance declines with excessive weight gain, making an extra carb load particularly destructive.

Metabolism is the body's process of converting substances ingested into other compounds. Sugar makes insulin levels go crazy, causing metabolism to shut down. This makes the body store more fat. Losing a lot of weight quickly means a large amount of lean tissue is lost, thus lowering the rate of metabolism. Losing weight without exercising could mean you are sacrificing muscle mass. Severely restrictive diets can reduce the metabolic rate by up to 30 percent. Strengthening exercises are critical to losing and maintaining weight. They help preserve muscle and bone, boosting your metabolism. Because muscle burns calories and fat doesn't, having a high level of lean muscle mass in your body and a low amount of fat means you will burn more calories, both during physical activity and when sitting in a chair, cooking dinner, or even while sleeping.

The energy used to keep the body alive (basal metabolism) accounts for 50–75 percent of daily caloric expenditure. Day-to-day activities burn 15–40 percent of calories. All physical activity burns calories, even walking to the fridge. The number of calories you burn generally depends on your body composition, metabolism, and food intake.

BEAUTY BYTES:

For help starting an exercise program, visit www.nutricise.com or www.4woman.org.

hired help

A certified nutrition expert or personal trainer can make the difference between dieting and working out day after day and not making any progress to achieving the shape of your dreams.

But just because your trainer looks like an Olympic medalist, it doesn't necessarily follow that they know anything about fitness and physiology. You have to check out their credentials before you sign up. Nutrition and fitness experts come with varying degrees of expertise, and many are certified in more than one area of specialization like weight management, weight training, or strength training. A registered dietitian is an expert in the science of nutrition and dietetics who is able to assist in evaluating nutritional information and supplementation, and translate it into practical application.

Determine what your needs are in terms of expertise, billing, flexibility, scheduling sessions, whether you are more comfortable with a man or a woman, frequency, and their rates. Ask for references, and get referrals from people who have used trainers and nutritional counselors before and were satisfied. Make sure they carry liability insurance. If you're under medical care, they should request a health screening from your doctor. Look for someone who makes you feel comfortable and motivates you, and whom you can get along with long-term.

A good place to start is at your gym. A trainer or fitness professional who works in a club will probably charge less per hour than one who works independently and comes to your home or office. To find a qualified food and nutrition expert log on to www.eatright.org, www.findanutritionist.com, or www.cdc.gov/niosh/diet/dietpac.html.

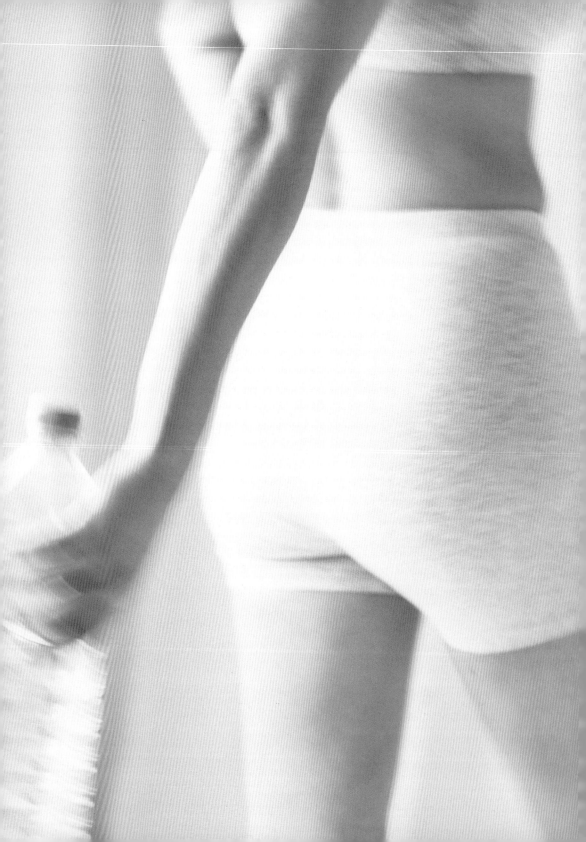

THE WAR ON DIMPLES

THE WAR ON DIMPLES

What does every woman over twenty have behind her? Cellulite. Although it's normal, the bad news is that there is no cure. An estimated 80-90 percent of women have some form of cellulite. The many causes begin with the usual suspects like genetics, stress, hormones, nutrition, caffeine, and smoking, and include excess fat, crash dieting, and rapid weight gain. Even sleeping pills, diuretics, and diet pills have been cited.

Cellulite lives in the subcutaneous layer of the skin. It varies in thickness and is laced with fat cells held in place by a network of fibers that cushions the muscles and organs. When all is well, waste products are removed and smooth curves result. When fats, fluids, and toxins are trapped deep in the skin, the tissue thickens and hardens, giving a dimpling effect. As we mature, the outer layer of the skin thins so the dimples become more obvious. The most cellulite-prone areas are the buttocks and thighs. Cellulite is most visible when you are standing. Topical agents, packs, wraps, massage, and ultrasound may offer temporary improvement, but there is no scientifically proven treatment that gets rid of it permanently. Reducing cellulite takes commitment and perseverance.

the bottom line

the bottom line

Cellulite is not necessarily a factor of body weight. All women know that you don't have to be heavy to have cellulite.

Although diet and lifestyle do affect cellulite formation, a large part of the problem is caused by the buildup of toxins and fat. Cellulite can affect any woman, regardless of size, weight, and body type. At some point, whether you're a size six or fourteen, if you're female, you're likely to see a skin pattern developing that looks a bit like quilting, and I don't mean the kind on Chanel bags. It starts on the back of your thighs, extends to the buttocks, and eventually travels to the dreaded saddlebags, the fronts of the thighs, buttocks, knees, and upper abdomen. This is cellulite and it has been known to reduce grown women to tears.

Estrogen production makes cellulite unique to women. Any fluctuation in hormone levels contributes to fat storage in the fat cells. As they expand to make room for extra fat, connective fibers are pulled down and fat cells bulge out. The skin is connected to the underlying structures by vertical fibrous bands, which act like buttons on a mattress, blocking the drainage of lymph fluid. As the trapped lymph fluid collects, the fibers get tighter and these areas of skin balloon up, causing dimpling of the skin. All of these factors create the dreaded "orange peel" effect.

Exercise is vital for achieving proper circulation, which combats cellulite formation and keeps your body toned. It also works to relieve tension, which stresses the muscles and causes the connective tissue that covers the muscles to seize up and block the tissues, preventing efficient waste elimination. Correct breathing and relaxation can ease your tension, oxygenate the body, and help with the body's natural purification process. The better your body functions, the more effectively it can eliminate the toxins that can cause cellulite.

eating patterns

A good way to start fighting cellulite is by detoxing, which means adding foods that are easiest for the body to break down, use, and get rid of, and subtracting anything that inhibits that process.

Drink eight to twelve cups of water a day to assist your body in getting rid of unwanted toxins and waste. The message is: Be good to your liver and it will metabolize fats more efficiently so you'll be less likely to develop the dreaded "C" word.

- **DOs** Fresh fruits • Vegetables • Whole-grain foods • Low fat • High fiber • Complex carbohydrates • Water

- **DON'Ts** Chocolate • Caffeine • Carbonated drinks • Alcohol • Sugar • Starches • Salt • Spices • Animal fats • Dairy • White flour • Processed foods • Fried foods

If your goal is to audition for *Baywatch*, you need to hire a nutritionist, personal chef, and trainer to design a diet and fitness program and keep you on it. It wouldn't hurt to stay out of bistros, bars, and cafés, either. Beware of diet saboteurs—people who may mean well but encourage you to treat yourself to dessert or bring you chocolates as a reward for losing a few pounds.

TOP TIP:
Avoid the "ine's"—caffeine, nicotine, wine, saccharine, margarine, and theobromine (chocolate).

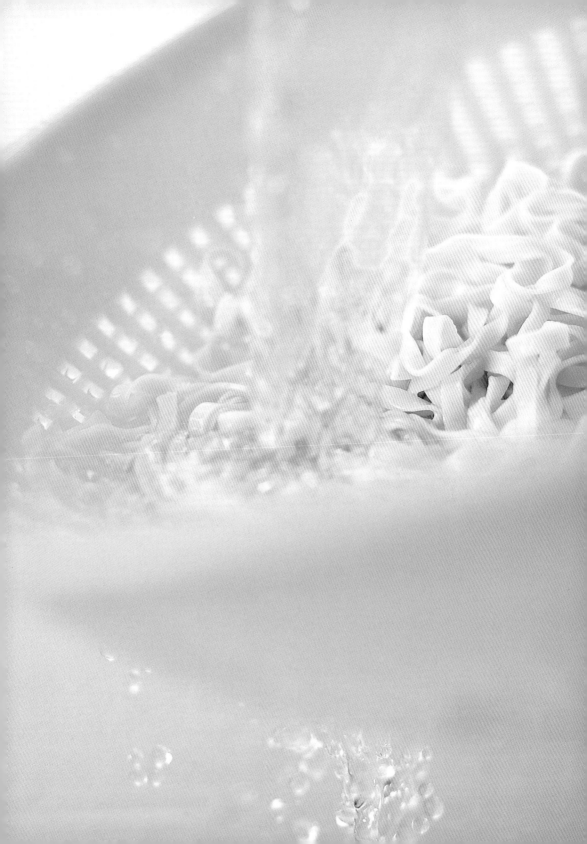

heavenly bodies

Cellulite may seem more ominous than regular fat, but it is just arranged differently. Weight loss and exercise will help minimize it, but you can still have lumps and bumps.

Kneading me

Massage techniques increase the circulation of blood and flow of lymph, a milky white fluid that carries impurities and waste out of the tissues. The oxygen capacity of the blood can increase by as much as 10–15 percent after vigorous massage. By manipulating the muscles, therapeutic massage stimulates the circulatory and lymphatic systems that break down fatty tissue. The lymph fluid does not circulate throughout the body as blood does, so it has to be moved around by putting pressure on the muscles so they contract. When you are still, the muscles contract less and consequently fail to stimulate lymph flow on their own.

The Swiss method of manual lymphatic drainage is widely used to speed up toxin elimination. It has an instant, but temporary, slimming effect. This technique can be used all over the body, from the face and neck down to the ankles, where fluid tends to settle. Deep tissue massage can also be useful in reducing cellulite by targeting areas that are difficult to stimulate with exercise, such as the inner knee and upper thigh. Simply massaging each leg in circular movements for a couple of minutes each day can help get rid of toxins.

BEAUTY BYTE:
For more about massage techniques, visit www.amtamassage.org.

Skin-fold rolling

Endermologie, the skin-fold rolling technology developed in France, temporarily reduces the appearance of cellulite. The operative word is "temporarily." Endermologie works by causing a swelling to the skin and underlying layers, which flattens out lumps and bumps. Endermologie is not the total answer; it is part of a multipronged approach to slimming and toning. A suction-roller device smooths the skin surface and stimulates circulation by eliminating toxins in the tissues.

Most women report feeling energized and relaxed after each session. Before the treatment, you slip into a sheer, white nylon leotard that runs from your neck to your ankles. Once you see yourself in this body stocking, you are sure to sign on for lifetime membership. Treatment begins with the therapist working on the back, then the calves, buttocks, thighs, feet, backs of the arms, and on to the neck and face. The focus is on cellulite-prone areas like the tummy, saddlebags, and front and backs of the thighs. After a series of forty-minute sessions once or twice per week for four to five months, be prepared for monthly maintenance or you can kiss your progress good-bye. Endermologie doesn't take away excess fat or any dress sizes. It works well as an adjunct to body liposuction to smooth and tone the skin once the fat cells are removed and has been shown to speed up the healing process. Combining Endermologie with ultrasound or sound waves may deliver longer-lasting results.

Thalassotherapy

Original thalassotherapy involves the use of seawater and sea air pumped from the ocean. Spa treatments are designed to re-create the benefits of the thalassotherapy experience. Ocean-derived ingredients include seaweed, sea minerals, and sea mud. Seaweed and algae saturated with mineral salts, trace elements, and amino acids are known for their rejuvenative properties and have long been used for weight loss and many ailments. With the properties of human plasma, seaweed absorbs nutrients of the sea, which transfer to the body when placed on the skin. Seaweeds are excellent sources of several vitamins, pantothenic acid, folic acid, niacin, and iodine. They are rich in minerals, especially potassium, calcium, magnesium, phosphorus, iron, zinc, and manganese. The treatments help encourage the body to eliminate waste materials, reduce excess water retention, and improve circulation.

Shrink wrap

Body wraps are commonly found on the menu of spa treatments for invigorating and detoxifying the skin. The body is usually swathed for up to an hour in mineral-rich mud, herbs, and/or seaweed-soaked cloths that aid in circulation and work to firm body contours. You can expect to be wrapped from your chest to your toes while lying on a thermal blanket to keep you warm and cozy. A technician then unwraps you. For the finishing touch, a body massage may be done to enhance circulation and encourage oxygen to flow to blocked tissues.

Dry brushing

Dry-skin brushing is a method used to remove dried, dead cells that block the pores of the skin. This allows the skin to breathe more easily and increases its ability to protect and eliminate the waste produced by metabolism. Dry brushing can also improve the skin's texture and appearance. It should be done using a natural-bristle body brush, a horsehair or nylon-bristle brush, or an exfoliating glove, before a bath or shower. Start with the lower limbs, arms, and back, then the front of the body, brushing the skin in an upward movement toward the heart, using a moderate pressure and short strokes. If you have a soft brush, the face can be done as well, using circular motions. The benefits of dry brushing are that it stimulates and increases blood circulation in all organs and tissues, especially capillaries near the skin. It aids the skin in ridding the system of toxins, placing less of a burden on the organs and nerve endings in the skin, and rejuvenates the entire nervous system. It can reduce cellulite deposits, tone and tighten the skin, increase resistance to colds, and improves overall health.

Mesotherapy

The technique of Mesotherapy was developed by Dr. Pistor in 1958 in France, to stimulate the mesoderm, or middle layer of the skin, using injections. The fibrous connective tissues, cartilage, bone, muscle, and fat make up the mesoderm layer. Natural plant extracts are used with a combination of agents like enzymes and nutrients to stimulate venous and lymph flow. Some doctors use a solution containing a vasodilator, which increases blood flow and stimulates lymph drainage, and a lipolytic agent to break down fat tissue. An anesthetic may also be used. Mesotherapy injections are given to improve the venous and lymphatic flow and also to break down the fat nodules. Extremely small needles are used, which just penetrate the body superficially, typically four to six millimeters.

The treatments are usually given once per week. As improvement is seen, the procedure may be repeated less frequently, such as once every two weeks or once a month. For long-term chronic conditions such as cellulite, at least fifteen sessions of Mesotherapy will be needed, and the process should be repeated as the cellulite returns.

Mesotherapy is done to avoid oral medications that have to go through the bloodstream to get to the area of the body that needs treatment. Droplets of the same medication are introduced through multiple microinjections at or around the problem spot, never too deep. Mesotherapy should be performed only by a medical doctor licensed to administer injections.

think yourself thin

Getting and staying svelte is also about using your brain. Your body sends you messages. If you fight them, diet plans can backfire.

Think before you open your mouth. Sometimes you'll lose weight more effectively if you pay attention to your body, rather than strictly adhering to a generic diet prescription. Consider what will satisfy your appetite at that particular moment. Stuffing yourself with celery sticks when you're craving a cookie can cause you to eat more than you want. Avoid turning your food into high anxiety by agonizing over every morsel you put into your mouth. Eat when you're hungry and stop when you feel full.

If you're starving, have a healthy snack at in the afternoon instead of waiting until dinner. Eat foods that make you feel good and give you energy instead of all that guilt. If you keep a bowl of fruit on your kitchen counter, you'll be more likely to reach for an apple than a bag of chips. Skipping breakfast won't spare you calories either. It can make you hungrier midmorning and at lunch. Spreading your food intake over the day is the best way to burn calories.

Determine a weight that is comfortable for you, and make it realistic. You may be better off stabilizing rather than losing more weight. A family history of obesity is not a reason to give up the battle. Your weight and the way your body stores fat is more closely linked with that of your mother, but genetics accounts for only about 25 percent of your risk of becoming plump. Making small changes that can be maintained over time is the real key.

Expert advice: Invest in a body fat monitor/scale that can estimate your body fat. To get the most accurate results, avoid moderate activity for twelve hours before stepping on the scale, don't eat for four hours, and don't have alcoholic drinks for forty-eight hours.

dos and don'ts for perfect curves

The secret is a combination of diet, exercise, and therapies. There are no quick fixes, including liposuction, which is not a cure for dimples. What you don't eat, drink, and do is more important than what you do.

- **DO** expect cellulite to become more noticeable with age as the connective tissue becomes stiffer and the skin holding the fat in place gets looser.

- **DO** drink six to eight glasses of water daily. Poor lymphatic flow, due to lack of physical activity and inadequate water intake, is a big contributor.

- **DO** avoid alcohol and soda. Even though cellulite may drive you to drink, wine, beer, and carbonated beverages keep you bloated.

- **DON'T** forget to exfoliate daily with AHA or BHA creams, and use a loofah or massage brush in the shower for stimulation and intense moisturizers to keep skin smooth.

- **DON'T** waste your money on electrostimulation treatments—join a gym, buy a dog to run in the park with, or hire a trainer.

- **DON'T** put much faith in anticellulite creams and gels to get rid of your dimpling. They will only temporarily firm and tone skin from the outside. The most effective of these treatments contain caffeine and retinol to tighten skin.

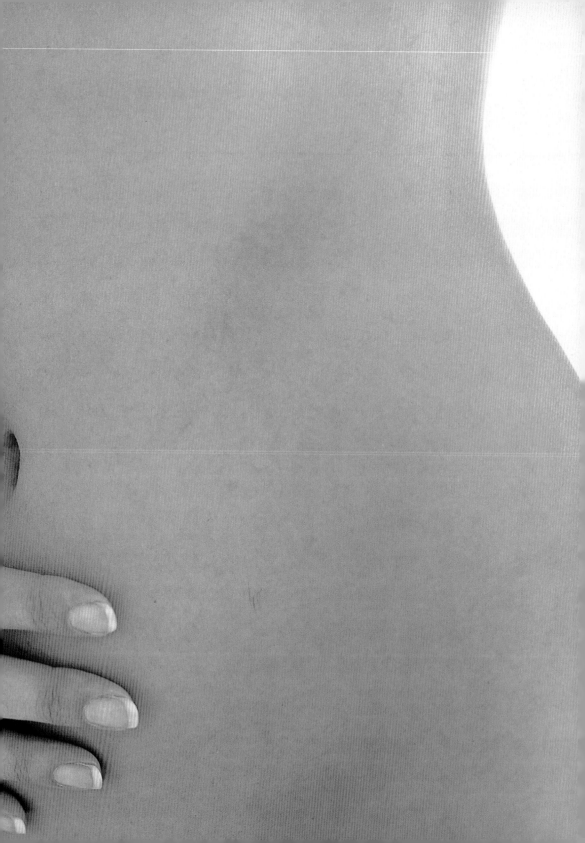

BODY CONTOURING

You go to the gym three times a week and watch what you eat, but you still feel like the rear end of a bus. Liposuction is an effective way to remove unsightly bulges, giving you an improved shape and contour. This explains why liposuction, or "lipoplasty," has long been the most popular cosmetic surgical procedure, worldwide. In 2001, according to the American Society for Aesthetic Plastic Surgery, 385,000 lipoplasties were performed in the United States alone. For women striving for a better body, getting rid of unwanted fat cells sounds like a dream come true. Picture this: You go to sleep with fatty bulges and when you awake, they're gone!

Adult fat cells are thought to be incapable of multiplying. As you gain weight, they expand, and as you lose weight, they contract, but the number and distribution stay the same. This accounts for why thin women still complain about localized fatty deposits that won't budge. Liposuction reduces your overall number of fat cells and changes your shape, so any future weight gain or loss won't be as noticeable in the areas that were treated. It can jump-start a serious weight loss and exercise program or be used to remove any resistant bulges.

outer limits

Liposuction is not a miracle cure—it can't give you the body of a supermodel. You can still gain weight after liposuction, but if you do, it will mostly be in areas not suctioned.

The ideal liposuction patient is at or close to normal weight. Most doctors will not perform liposuction on patients who are twenty-eight pounds or more overweight, or over 30 percent more than their ideal body weight. If you're just fourteen pounds away from a size that is acceptable to you, lose some weight before surgery and more after. If you put on a few pounds after lipo, you'll blow your investment. If you lose some, your result will look that much better. It is not uncommon to have a small touch-up procedure six months later.

These procedures are for anyone who cannot obtain the trim and contoured look that they are after with diet and exercise, and possess good skin elasticity. There are limits as to how many areas can be operated on and how much fat can be removed, based on your size, weight, and tolerance to surgery. With new techniques, amounts of five to ten pounds of fat and fluids can be removed at one stage. If there are several areas you want suctioned, you can easily reach that level. If there is too much for one stage, the surgeon may suggest that you lose weight before having liposuction. When skin elasticity is not ideal, a staged procedure is a good solution. The liposuction would be done first, and if you don't get enough skin contraction, then skin excision and internal tightening can be done at a later date, as in a tummy tuck or a thigh lift. In certain cases, up to ten to twenty pounds of fat may be suctioned, which is categorized as large volume lipoplasty, and is considered far more risky.

YES, IT CAN

- Remove fat deposits
- Change your shape
- Take out fat from beneath the skin

NO, IT CAN'T

- Cure cellulite
- Tighten loose skin
- Take out fat from underneath muscles

Before having liposuction, your cosmetic surgeon should discuss your lifestyle, fitness level, and body-weight fluctuations. If you have a history of an eating disorder like bulimia, anorexia, or binge eating, or have been on prescription weight-control medications, tell your surgeon in advance. Some areas of the body have fatty deposits that tend to stick around no matter how much you starve yourself or how many miles you jog, sit-ups you do, or laps you swim. Fat deposits that don't respond to the usual exercise and diet regimes are ideal targets for liposuction. If you are only overweight in certain areas of your body, for example, you have saddlebags, you would have to lose a large amount of weight in order to shrink the size of your thighs. The weight will come off from everywhere, including the breasts and face, and not just directly where you need it most. The beauty of liposuction surgery is that it will just focus on your chosen areas.

After liposuction there are still fat cells in the areas that were suctioned, so those body parts are not off limits. The good news is that if you do gain fat in areas of the body that weren't your primary trouble spots, it is usually very responsive to diet and exercise. For example, if you have liposuction on your stomach and you gain seven pounds afterward, it may show up on your hips instead. When you lose that weight, it will go quicker from the hips because it was the last place the fat was gained.

the art of liposuction

Liposuction has come a long way since its introduction in the mid-1970s. Modern techniques are vastly improved for women who want to make their fat cells history.

Typically, women in their twenties and thirties, go for liposuction of their inner and outer thighs and knees. In the forties and fifties, in addition to the thighs, the abdomen, hips, waist, and upper back become popular due to gaining weight with each pregnancy. Extra weight gained in your perimenopausal years tends to settle around your midsection. By age sixty, the hips and bottom spread, and liposuction procedures give way to body lifts as skin thins and elasticity is lost.

The procedure is very straightforward. The surgeon uses cannulas—hollow, tubular instruments with holes at one end to trap the fat. The cannula is attached to suction tubing through which the excess fat is evacuated. These instruments come in various shapes, lengths, and sizes depending on the thickness and location of the fat. They have highly polished surfaces to slip through the fatty tissues with minimum friction or damage, so there is less bruising. The instruments are typically blunt-tipped to prevent cutting through the skin, and fat is suctioned out through strategically placed holes at the tip. Traditional liposuction relies on the mechanical disruption of fat cells by the movement of the cannula and the vacuum of the suction pump. Tiny incisions are made at the sites where fat is to be removed, and a wetting solution is infused to provide a numbing effect, reduce bleeding, and improve fat extraction. Cannulas are inserted under the skin, moved in a back-and-forth and crisscross fashion within the fat, then the fat is vacuumed away. The size of the cannulas used can affect the smoothness of the skin after liposuction. The use of large cannulas tends to create irregularities more often than cannulas of less than three millimeters in diameter.

The output of fat is measured and the patient is checked for symmetry, although most of us have one side that is naturally slightly fuller than the other. The procedure is completed when a safe level of fat removal is achieved. You are then monitored closely to make sure you have received enough fluid hydration and are able to urinate without difficulty. After tumescent liposuction, some blood-tinged local anesthetic solution remains under the skin. This excess fluid is either slowly absorbed into the bloodstream or rapidly removed by draining through skin incisions. Rapid drainage reduces postoperative pain, swelling, and bruising. Surgery can be performed in a hospital or at an accredited clinic. For larger procedures, staying in the hospital or clinic overnight may be recommended.

New studies have shown that liposuction may provide additional health benefits for some women. A dramatic reduction in body weight can be useful as a stepping-stone to long-term weight loss. Large-volume liposuction (the removal of more than ten pounds or five quarts of fat) may also lead to a lowering of blood pressure and insulin levels in some women who are more than fifty pounds above their ideal weight. Strict post-op monitoring is vital after aggressive liposuction procedures.

TOP TIP:
The larger the volume of fat and fluids removed from the body, the more risky the procedure becomes and the longer the recovery is likely to be.

fat traps

Technological advances in liposuction techniques have greatly improved the results and made it safer, faster, and more effective.

A major benefit of liposuction is that the scars left are tiny, less than half an inch. Small, slitlike scars can be placed in hidden areas like the belly button, the crease under the buttocks, and inside the knee. These generally heal well and are rarely evident, even in the teeniest thong.

A warmed, diluted sterile solution containing lidocaine, epinephrine, and intravenous fluid is injected into the area to be treated. As the liquid enters the fat, it becomes swollen, firm, and blanched. The expanded fat compartments allow the liposuction cannula to travel smoothly beneath the skin as the fat is removed. Saline softens the fat, adrenaline decreases the bruising, and the anesthetic provides pain relief. For small amounts of fat, tumescent solution may be the only anesthetic given. The solution can also be supplemented with sedatives to relax you during the procedure. General anesthesia may be used for larger procedures involving multiple areas.

Specific risks include rare complications like pulmonary edema—fluid in the lungs—which may occur if too much fluid is administered, and lidocaine toxicity, which can occur if there is too much lidocaine in the solution. If too much solution is injected, there is a risk of drowning in fluids. Overworking the heart is a possible consequence. There is also the possibility of causing a fat embolism, which is when a piece of fat travels into the bloodstream. Generally, the greater the volume of fat and fluids removed, the higher the chances of having a complication.

Internal ultrasound: Ultrasonic sound waves, like shock waves, are transmitted into the fatty tissues from the tip of a fine probe. Ultrasonic energy is used to liquefy or melt the fat, which is then removed using a cannula and a low-pressure vacuum. Ultrasonic liposuction is often used for large volumes and multiple areas and is good for areas where the deep fat is thicker and harder to get out; e.g., back rolls and upper abdomen. It is usually combined with traditional liposuction when both the deeper and the more superficial fat is being removed. When previous liposuction has been done, it may be useful to soften the resulting scar tissue to make it easier for the surgeon to remove the fat. Some patients report a slight burning sensation after surgery.

External ultrasound: Ultrasonic energy is used in lower frequencies to soften fat deposits and smooth out bumps on the skin's surface. It is also used after liposuction to break up the hard spots and lumpiness, especially on the tummy.

Vaser: This new ultrasound technology utilizes bursts of ultrasonic energy to break up fat cells for removal. Smaller, more delicate probes are used to increase the surgeon's precision and the safety of the procedure.

Power trip

In 1998, the use of power was introduced to fat-sucking methods. The cannulas used are motor-driven, so they vibrate as they work, which makes removing fat easier and faster for the surgeon. The reciprocating frequency provides enough energy through the tip of the instruments to glide through fatty tissue. Since less physical exertion is required, many surgeons report that they can get better results and remove more fat. Postoperative pain, bruising, and swelling may also be reduced with this method.

liposculpture

Liposculpture is a superficial variation on liposuction whereby smaller amounts of fat are removed and reinjected to create improved contour.

Liposculpture, also called syringe liposculpture, was introduced in the mid-1980s. It uses fine instruments to remove small amounts of fat to define features, accentuate muscles, and sharpen the appearance of the neck, cheeks, abdomen, buttocks, calves, and ankles. Superficial liposuction techniques remove tiny bits of fat just under the surface of the skin, and fat injections may be used to fill in contour defects. Some cosmetic surgeons gently break down adhesions and cellulite deposits by cutting through the fibrous tissues with *V*-shaped instruments. This technique smooths out irregularities. Since liposuction became popular, surgeons have used progressively smaller instruments, so it is now a more delicate procedure. The really good surgeons can reshape your contours in a very subtle way, causing minimal trauma to the tissue.

TOP TIP:
Look at your body naked in a full-length mirror. Evaluate each part separately—the upper abdomen, lower abdomen, legs, etc. To achieve the most attractive curves possible, focus on the areas you would benefit most from having recontoured. For example, if your thighs bulge, liposuctioning just one part, like the outer portion, may make the inner thighs or hips look too large in comparison.

body parts

Almost any body part can be suctioned for better contour and reduced volume, from the face all the way down to the ankles.

The most popular areas for women are the abdomen, inner and outer thighs, hips, flanks, and knees. The trend is to treat areas of the body circumferentially, instead of removing fat deposits from selected spots. Sections like the abdomen, hips, waist, and all around the thighs and knees, and upper arms, are combined to maximize the potential for skin to shrink afterward. It is not rare to have liposuction done in stages; for example, the lower body in one go and the trunk later. Liposuction can even be used to reduce large breasts in women whose breasts have a lot of fatty tissue.

Ab flab

Generally speaking, the springier your skin is, the better liposuction works. If your greatest concern is flabby skin due to pregnancy, aging, or yo-yo dieting, liposuction can actually make it look worse. Some fatty areas are less forgiving to major fat removal than others and more often lead to sagging skin; for example, upper arms, inner thighs, knees, abdomen, and the neck, in women. If your ultimate goal is to be taut and supertrim from the waist down, a tummy tuck, thigh lift, or lower body lift are the only viable options. These involve tightening underlying muscles and removing and redraping excess skin. Unfortunately, they leave significant scarring and the recovery period is longer, but the results can be amazing.

The right to bare arms

Some call them "bat wings"—those dreaded flabby arms can really hurt someone if they swing when you wave good-bye. Along with inner thighs, upper arms are the pet hate of more women than we can count. If you're longing to go sleeveless, read on. Intensive upper extremity exercises with weight training help greatly, but after a certain age or if gravity has taken a toll on the thin skin of the arms, improvement won't be dramatic or quick. If you have good, elastic skin, liposuction can be the answer to your prayers. Plastic surgeons can recontour the upper arm by taking out fat through tiny incisions around the elbow. You won't end up with perfectly toned, defined arms, but you may be able to go sleeveless with pride. The skin contracts to a better shape after about three weeks, when the bruising and most of the swelling has gone. After about three months, you can see the final contour change.

Rubber tires

Women have a layer of fat stored on their abdomen. The pelvic region swells from monthly bloating, and the body adapts by outwardly stretching these muscles. Over time, the lower tummy softens up and creates a bulge. Particularly in women who have had children and those in the perimenopausal range (from the forties onward), fat deposits tend to accumulate in the middle section of the body. If you can't remember the last time you had a waist and your hips seem to have a mind of their own, liposuction may be able to help bring you back into belt-donning shape. The upper and lower tummy, waist, hips, and flanks can be suctioned to reduce girth. It is not a substitute for a full tummy tuck or abdominoplasty, but most women in reasonably good health and firmness can get some skin shrinkage. If it is a washboard stomach you crave, then a more invasive surgery, which tightens the muscles and removes excess skin, is in order.

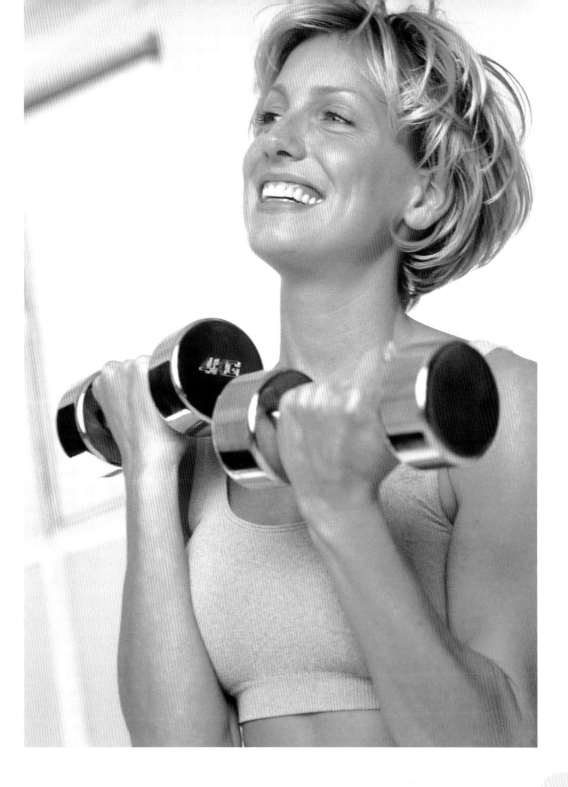

Thigh zone

The abdomen, buttocks, and thighs are undoubtedly the "Bermuda Triangle" for women. The buttocks are the first part to lose shape due to gravity. As muscles weaken, they gradually become unable to support the fat. What one woman calls her buttocks, a cosmetic surgeon might refer to as her "lateral thighs" or "banana rolls"—the fold of skin and fat just below the buttock crease. Another issue for women is how each body part flows into the next. For example, how the buttocks are connected to the hips and outer thighs. The topic of rear ends is about contour and proportions; i.e., the transition from the trunk to the buttocks should be smooth and appear as though they belong to the rest of your body, instead of having a life of their own.

Improving the backside involves taking out and putting in fat. Liposuction can be done for hips, thighs, and banana rolls, but is rarely recommended near the buttock crease because removing the fat can actually increase sagging. The best candidates are women who are a size eight on top and a twelve below. If you have a small backside with protruding thighs, recontouring only the buttocks may make the thighs look that much bigger. They are usually done as a set. Fat from other body parts can be sucked out and injected back to smooth out your gluteus maximus, fill out dents, and add curves. If you're waifish everywhere else, you may be stuck with a flat rear.

TOP TIP:
If you have had scoliosis or any type of hip injury, one side may appear higher than the other.

The good news is that the outer thighs usually respond very well to liposuction and can give you a posterior view to be proud of even in your tightest-fitting jeans.

A leg up

Getting your legs fit to bare can be high maintenance. Flabby knees are the bane of any woman's existence, and all the crunches and squats on earth won't make them go away significantly if that is your problem spot. Many women think they have Miss Piggy knees, when, in fact, it is their joints that make their knees look large and not fat at all. Liposuction can be used to delicately recontour legs from the ankles, calves, and knees up to the inner and outer thighs, taking inches off the circumference of the leg. Fatty deposits can, in many cases, be suctioned away from the inner portion of the knees. The flabby pouches on the front of the knees are not really ideal for reduction by liposuction. Calves are tricky because they are often largely muscle, but suctioning even small amounts can make a big difference to the overall shape.

Liposuction of the legs takes longer than other areas to fully settle down, because swelling tends to travel downward and rest below the knee. This is one procedure that is usually best left for colder months when you can easily cover up bruising and swelling by wearing trousers, long skirts, and opaque tights. Scars are hidden and tiny, so they won't give your secret away, and support hose will help keep swelling to a minimum.

Heavy legs are also an inherited trait. If your mother or grandmother carried their weight in the thighs to the ankles, the chances are that you will, too.

TOP TIP:

DON'T sit with your legs crossed with one thigh on top of the other. This impedes blood flow and can increase thigh size as waste fluids build up in the legs, causing aches, pains, and cramps.

risks and recovery

Speedy healing has made the popularity of liposuction soar. You can be back at work after a long weekend. In a couple of weeks, you'll be ready for bikini season.

Generally, patients have significant swelling for two days following the procedure, but this rapidly subsides, and resolves quickly over the next few weeks. You should look good after three weeks and continue to improve over the next three to six months. Bruising is usually minimal and showering is permitted after two days. Many women return to work or some activity within two to four days for small liposuctions, ten to fourteen days for more extensive procedures. Many resume an exercise program in two weeks. Post-op pain is minimal, especially with an expertly administered anesthetic. You will see your new shape best after three weeks, when most of the swelling has subsided. After six months, the final contour will be visible. If you are having thighs, knees, or ankles done, keeping your legs elevated will reduce the swelling faster.

After surgery, a compression garment will be applied that keeps swelling to a minimum. Most women feel better with some compression and wear the girdle or support hose for longer. Antiembolism boots are often used during surgery to prevent a blood clot from forming in the deep veins of the pelvis or legs. The risk of a seroma—an oozing or pooling of clear serum—is possible in certain areas, like the abdomen, after ultrasound techniques have been used. In these cases, the surgeon may drain the excess fluid to relieve pressure. The other risks apply to an surgical procedure and include infection, bleeding, skin loss, and nerve damage. All of these are rare. Generally, the greater the volume of fat and fluids removed, the higher the chances of having a problem.

honey, I shrunk

After liposuction, most women find that they have a better shape with fewer bulges. Clothes that were snug around the hips and thighs will flow nicely without pulling and stretching.

- You will weigh more right after liposuction than before surgery. Your face, feet, and hands will swell up from all the fluids pumped into you.

- Swelling travels down like everything else, so don't be surprised if you're puffy and bruised in places you didn't have suctioned.

- Warm, aromatic baths infused with lavender and rosemary can soothe and relax sore body parts.

- Use petroleum jelly, bacitracin, or vitamin E oil to keep incisions soft and to keep scabs from forming. Don't pick at scabs, as they will take longer to heal and potentially scar.

- You may find that you itch like mad and your skin is dry and flaky. Try a rich body lotion, a loofah, and oatmeal baths.

- Avoid crash diets and appetite suppressants or diet drugs for at least two weeks after surgery. You need nourishment and lots of water, juices, and sports drinks in order to get back to optimum health.

- Don't ditch your old wardrobe or go clothes shopping for at least six weeks after liposuction. You will still be shrinking and won't have seen your final result yet.

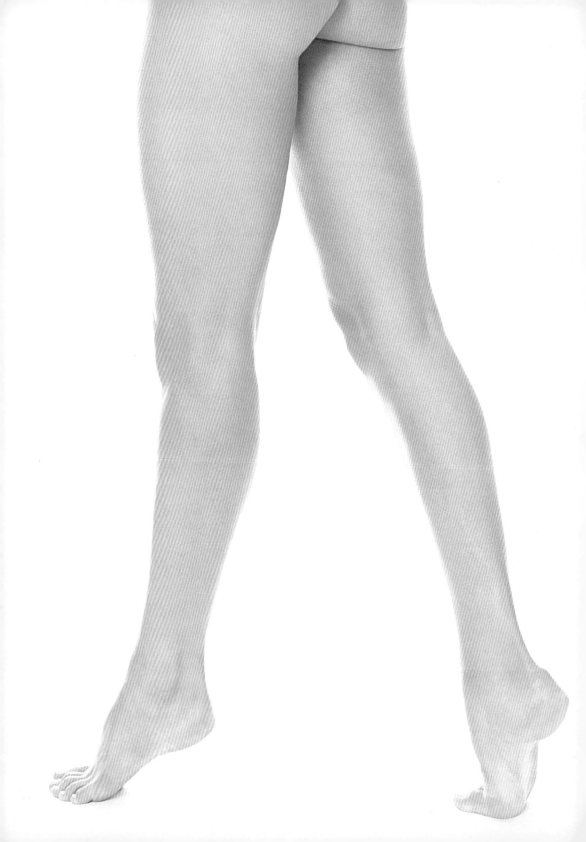

SKINNY SURGERY

SKINNY SURGERY

The last frontier in figure reshaping is the most radical. If you've done all you can at the gym and the dinner table, there are still several options left to recontour your body back into beautiful form. These should be considered as the last resort, after you have done your part.

If your skin tone is good, you are best served by liposuction. However, if you have an abundance of loose skin on the abdomen or thighs, or have lost a great deal of weight that has left you with a slimmer, but looser, body, liposuction won't do the job and may make your ripples look worse. When the degree of skin excess is too severe to be overcome by exercise alone, skin removal, in the form of a body lift, is needed. Stand in front of a full-length mirror, grab ahold of some loose skin and pull up. Voilà, that's basically what a body lift can do.

If you are severely obese and have several dress sizes to lose to get you to the shape you want, gastric surgery may be suggested to restrict your food intake so you can lose a lot of weight safely. None of these procedures are quick fixes, and they are not ideal for everybody.

bariatric surgery

Gastrointestinal surgery for obesity helps to restrict food intake by closing off parts of the stomach to make it smaller, or by limiting the absorption of ingested foods.

Since its introduction in 1954, bariatric surgery has become increasingly popular. In 2002, 75,000 people had these operations in the United States alone. Gastrointestinal surgery may be recommended for people who are one hundred pounds or more overweight and is reserved for those who cannot lose weight by traditional means or who suffer from serious obesity-related health problems. To be eligible, you have to be morbidly obese, or have a body mass index of forty or above (see page 76).

The first operation that was widely used for severe obesity was the intestinal bypass, which produced weight loss by causing malabsorption. The concept was that if large amounts of food were eaten, they would be poorly digested or passed along too fast for the body to absorb the calories, but the side effects included a loss of essential nutrients and pain.

The Roux-en-Y: The stomach is separated and a very small pouch is created through stapling or banding to curtail food intake. A *Y*-shaped section of the small intestine is redirected to the pouch with a narrow opening, bypassing the first and second sections of the intestine to limit food absorption. The procedure requires three days in hospital and a one to three week recovery. Eighty percent of patients lose at least half their excess weight.

Restrictive surgery also serves to reduce food intake but differs from malabsorptive surgery in that it does not interfere with the digestive process.

Vertical Banded Gastroplasty: This less invasive method limits food intake by creating a small pouch in the upper stomach. The pouch fills quickly and empties slowly, producing a feeling of fullness. Overeating will result in pain or vomiting and will stretch the pouch. Only half of patients lose at least 50 percent of their excess weight. This procedure is performed as a day surgery and recovery takes seven to ten days.

LAP-BAND adjustable gastric banding system: In this newer method used to limit food intake, a constricting ring is placed completely around the upper end of the stomach just below the junction of the stomach and the esophagus, creating an hourglass effect. No cutting or stapling of the stomach is required, the outlet size is adjustable, and the band is easily removed for restoration of normal stomach anatomy. At present, there are only two devices on the market, and the Lap-Band is only freely available in the United States, having been approved for use by the FDA.

These procedures can now be done laparoscopically via a fiber-optic tube inserted through small incisions in the abdominal wall. As in other treatments for obesity, the best results are achieved with healthy eating behaviors and regular physical activity. Having the surgery is not a license to pig out, and compulsive overeaters who don't take charge of their eating disorder can still gain weight after surgery. For more information on bariatric surgery, log on to www.asbsorg and www.naaso.org.

body lifts

If sagging and dragging are the problem, a lift may be the only answer. Body lifts are usually performed in tandem with liposuction.

Body lifts are ideal for women who have had a significant weight loss and are left with unsightly loose pouches of excess skin. It is the most invasive, yet the most effective technique to restore firm, youthful contours to the body. If you look in the mirror naked and pull up the saggy skin of your hips to stretch out your upper thighs and abdominal area, you can transform the way your body looks. Body lifts essentially do the same thing. A toned body is firm and healthy, with a strong network of layers of muscle fibers and fatty tissues underneath the skin. Lower body lifts attack the thighs, buttocks, abdomen, waist, and hips all in one stage. The added benefits are an overall improvement in dimpling and cellulite, as well as the general elevation of a woman's private parts to a more youthful status.

The good news is a body lift can give you the body of a twenty-year-old. The not-so-good news is that the scars are extensive and recovery is longer than most other cosmetic surgical procedures, about three weeks.

The body-lift procedure involves the removal of excess skin and fat. The fat is lifted off the muscle and the hanging skin is elevated and tacked into a higher position. Stitches are placed in layers to the deeper structures below and attached to hold the fat and skin securely in place. Ideally, body lifting procedures should be undertaken once you have lost your weight and kept it off long term. Often, multiple stages are required if there are many areas of loose, hanging skin; for example, the lower torso, breasts and arms, and inner thighs and knees. The idea behind the body lift is to first use liposuction to contour the underlying fat, smooth it out, then lift the looseness around it.

If you have had previous liposuction and now have an unevenness or irregularities, the next step would be a skin-tightening procedure. If you can pinch up the skin and it feels thin or loose, you may be a candidate. For any surgery involving wide incisions, smokers should be very cautious, as nicotine interferes with wound healing and can increase the risks of infection and poor scars.

Lower Body

The lower body lift tightens and lifts the hips, buttocks, and outer thighs. It requires an incision around the entire circumference of the abdominal area to remove flabby skin and lift the flank, thigh, and buttocks areas. The incision can usually be placed discreetly within standard or high-cut bikini lines. The result of the procedure is a tightened lower back, flank, and abdominal skin and removal of cellulite in these areas. Lower body lifts are considered among the most invasive of all cosmetic surgery procedures, the recovery is lengthy, and scarring is not for the squeamish. If inner thighs and saggy knees are the problem, a medial or inner thigh lift is required. For this a horizontal incision is generally placed in the groin area and excess skin is lifted and removed. These scars can drop over time, but there is no other surgery to tighten this area.

Upper Body

Some areas of fat deposits are less forgiving to major fat removal than others, and more often lead to sagging skin; for example, upper arms and inner thighs in women are thinner-skinned areas and don't always contract well past the age of forty. For flabby upper arms that don't respond to liposuction alone, an arm lift can be done, which involves a linear incision on the underside of the upper arm from the elbow to the armpit.

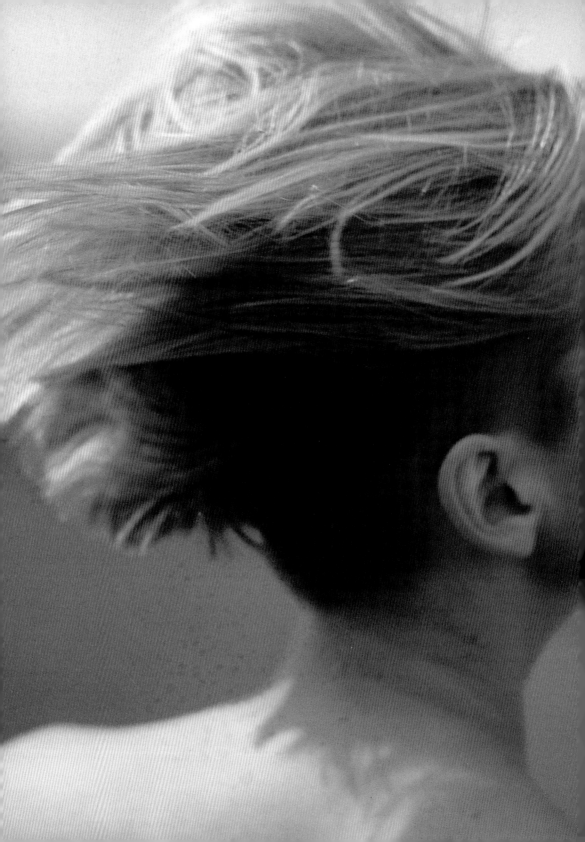

HAIR AFFAIR

HAIR AFFAIR

Never underestimate the power of great hair. It is the frame around your face, the finishing touch to your total look. It is an essential part of your image and a great accessory. It's one of the first things you notice about a person.

A good hairstyle can be the ultimate fashion statement. Hairstyles change every season, but whatever the look, thick is always in. Both women and men tend to be most attracted to a head of hair that is dense, long, and a good color. The goal is shine, softness, strength, and "stylability," which are key indicators of healthy hair and what every woman craves.

The expression "bad hair day" has become a part of our vernacular. Its closest translation: If your hair doesn't look good, you don't look good. Thin, limp, or stringy hair makes you feel like a plain Jane. How you wear your hair says a lot about you. Gorgeous hair connotes real beauty and a new hairstyle is the quickest path to reinventing yourself. Faking it can be the next best thing.

clean regime

Just like your face, your hair needs a cleansing ritual for the morning, the evening, and emergencies. These may change with the seasons.

Great-looking hair starts in the shower. Go gently on your follicles to maintain each strand for as long as you can and to keep them bouncy. Overcleansing, pulling and tugging, and too much styling and fixing can weaken hair and make it brittle. Many shampoo bottles have directions that instruct you to shampoo and rinse twice. The idea is that the first removes dirt, oil, and product buildup and the second helps add volume, as well as providing a backup in case the first shampoo didn't get your hair clean enough. However, for dry or brittle hair, one shampoo may be enough.

The presence of airborne pollutants and holes in the ozone layer, and the use of steam heat, hot rollers, and blow-dryers means your hair tends to attract dust and dirt. For some women, daily washing with a shampoo formulated to restore balance to the hair and scalp is a necessity. Others are happy to skip a day or two. For short hair, daily washing is usually needed. Every other day for longer hair may be suitable, especially since the time involved to dry and style can be more than you can manage. Washing hair more than once a day is not necessary or recommended. The natural oils your hair produces each day provide thickness and shine that you don't want to strip away by overwashing.

shampoo selection

Selecting the right products for your hair type and condition will help you make the most of it. Start with the basics and add as needed. Your hair may grow tired of a product before you do.

Shampoos for colored, permed, or processed hair: Chemically processed hair needs special formulas that won't strip color and contain ingredients that are gentle and moisturizing.

Highlighting or color-enhancing shampoos: Designed to prevent color from fading, these add tone and extend the life of your highlights. They add shine to gray hair and help reduce yellow. They are also good to use after a permanent, as the peroxide in neutralizers can lighten the color of your hair.

Clarifying shampoos: These contain an acidic ingredient, such as lemon juice or vinegar, to cut through residue built up by styling products. Use these before you color, perm, or relax your hair to allow the treatment to be absorbed better and go on more evenly. They are too drying to use every day; once or twice a week is enough. Overuse can cause excess stripping of the natural oils.

Volumizing or body-building shampoo: These contain proteins that bond to the hair to add volume. Use them sparingly, as overuse may build up residue. For fine hair, alternate with a regular shampoo. Look for ingredients like "dimethicone copolyol"; a silicon derivative that helps to build volume in hair.

conditioner choices

Conditioners make the hair smoother and add body and shine, but there is a fine line between the right amount of conditioner and too much.

Conditioners are usually made of large molecules that literally stick to the outside of the hair and make combing easier, which prevents the hair from twisting and breaking. Hair tangles when the cuticle doesn't lie flat and the hairs can't slide past one another with ease. Because they coat the hair, conditioners make it look shiny and protect it from damage from the environment and styling tools. They usually contain silicone and moisture-producing substances like ceramides and complex lipids that smooth over hair and can reduce frizz and static electricity.

Although conditioners can add thickness and volume to thin and thinning hair, overconditioning may cause hair to look greasy. It can cause the cuticle layer of the hair to lift, making it brittle. Whether you use conditioner or not depends on your hair. For thin hair, use only lightweight, rinse-out conditioners. Volumizers with ingredients like keratin, collagen, and hydrolyzed proteins help to plump up strands for fuller-looking hair. Chemically processed hair needs conditioner to counteract the drying and damaging effects of the dyes and peroxides.

Most of us don't give conditioners time to work. Don't rinse out too soon before the conditioner has had a chance to seep into the hair. Wait at least five minutes.

TOP TIP:
Conditioners should be at a low pH of 4.0 to 4.5 to maintain the protein in the hair.

Daily conditioners

Dry hair

Leave-in conditioners

These treatments are usually applied to towel-dried hair. They coat the hair, making it heavier and weighing it down. Some formulas have UV protection built in to protect hair from sun, wind, and heat.

Dry and damaged hair

Deep conditioners

Hot oils

They include proteins and moisturizing ingredients to repair split ends and brittleness. They are usually left on for ten to thirty minutes and rinsed out thoroughly. Massage a few drops directly into the scalp every two to four weeks. Apply lightly to avoid overgreasing.

Fine and curly hair

Thickening serums

Detanglers

Proteins and polymers are bound to the hair shaft, making hair fuller. Apply to wet hair before styling. These work well as a substitute for conditioner on both fine and curly hair. Choose a light formula and rinse out thoroughly before combing hair.

Most hair types

Rinse-out conditioners

All-in-one shampoo/conditioners

These increase shine, smooth the hair cuticle, soften the hair, and reduce static. They are used after shampooing and should be rinsed out thoroughly. Shampoo/conditioner combos tend to leave a residue that builds up quickly and weighs hair down. They should never be used on oily hair. Best reserved for travel.

the white stuff

The condition of your scalp can provide a useful clue to the health of your hair. A healthy scalp provides a strong foundation for a gorgeous, shiny head of hair.

Part your hair in a place near the crown where you can see it in the mirror. Run a fine-tooth comb gently across the scalp. See how much flaking you pick up. Some occasional flaking is normal and doesn't necessarily mean you have dandruff. It could be a form of dermatitis or eczema. Dandruff is characterized by a dry, itchy scalp and white flakes that show up on your shoulders, especially when you're wearing dark colors. Dandruff is a normal shedding of skin, and is actually a form of seborrhea that is more common in men than in women. The exact cause is unknown but contributing factors can include stress, sweating, and hormones.

Dandruff can be present in dry or oily scalps, but is more common in oily skin types. The key to controlling dandruff is to remove the flakes as soon as they appear by frequent washing with a medicated shampoo, which not only removes the dandruff but also cuts down on the rate of shedding. For most sufferers, dandruff is a lifetime condition that can be controlled by using the right shampoo.

TOP TIP:
African and black women tend to have drier hair, which is likely to attract flakes. Daily shampooing may not be necessary. Massage the scalp to stimulate your natural oils. A light-textured oil can be used on the scalp, or ask your doctor about using a shampoo that contains a steroid.

Over-the-counter medicated shampoos usually contain coal tar, salicylic acid (beta hydroxy acid), selenium sulfide, or zinc pyrithione. Prescription strength sulfur, ketoconazole, and topical steroids may also be used. If your hair is processed, avoid products with selenium sulfide or sulfur.

Severe dandruff, where flakes are oilier and more yellowish than usual and the scalp is inflamed, might be seborrheic dermatitis, which requires treatment from a doctor. Use every day until your dandruff disappears. For maintenance, use medicated shampoos only as needed to avoid drying out your hair. Use a shampoo and conditioner for dry hair the rest of the time.

- **DON'T** use heavy conditioners and styling products designed to coat the hair, as they can prevent the natural shedding of the scalp. This may cause a buildup of flakes.

- **DO** switch to a gentler product, which may reduce flaking if your scalp is reacting to a harsh ingredient in your shampoo.

- **DO** use a clarifying shampoo, which may reduce product buildup and help to clear the scalp of flakes.

- **DO** use tea tree oil, which can be helpful as an antiseptic.

- **DO** give yourself regular scalp massages.

- **DO** try to avoid centrally heated rooms as dry scalp conditions can be aggravated by a lack of moisture in the air.

oil spills

Hair has natural oils secreted from the sebaceous glands to protect hair and keep it shiny. Oily hair may be greasy at the scalp, but dull and dry at the ends.

Fine, thin hair is the most prone to looking oily and limp. Wash hair daily with a mild shampoo that does not contain a conditioner so it leaves the least amount of residue. Formulas specifically for oily hair and clarifying shampoos work well. Use only a very light conditioner or a diluted formula on the ends only and rinse out thoroughly.

Greasy hair needs conditioning, too, it just needs less. Avoid products containing silicone, mineral oils, and lanolin, which coat the hair, weigh it down, and make the strands lie flat against the scalp. If your hair has become stringy by midday, spritz water on it and comb through to remove and redistribute oils. The goal is to avoid stripping away all its natural oils.

In humid weather, you may shower and wash your hair more often, especially if oily. Switch to a gentle shampoo for frequent use. If you sweat a lot when exercising, shampoo after your workout.

It is time to switch shampoos if:

- You like your hair better the morning after you've washed it.
- Your hair feels weighed down and you feel the need to rinse it more.
- Your hair is hard to detangle or style.
- Your hair doesn't look shiny.
- Sudsing no longer gives you a rich lather.

On rainy days, hair attracts moisture, which can make it go wild and very elastic. Fix it with a finishing spray to keep it where you want it.

Oil overdrive

Excess oil means your sebaceous glands are in overdrive. The waxy oil these glands produce not only gives hair a greasy appearance but also builds up on the scalp. When sebum hardens, it blocks blood flow and starves the roots embedded in the scalp. The roots are weakened and hair loss can occur. Excess oil makes your head a magnet for dirt, sometimes giving it the appearance of a string mop.

Scalp checkup: Part your hair at the crown and blot your scalp with a soft white paper tissue. If any residue shows, you have an oily scalp.

Magic hands

Nothing beats a great massage to stimulate blood flow to the scalp, keep your hair in peak condition, and relax you from your head to your toes. Massage has not been scientifically proved to stimulate new hair growth, however.

Begin by wetting your hair. Choose one of the natural ingredients listed below, depending on the condition of your scalp. Add a splash to some warm mineral water to make a solution. Drizzle the mixture through your hair, massaging as you go.

Dry or tight scalp: Warm almond oil, sesame oil, or a light olive oil.
Greasy scalp: Astringents like witch hazel, lemon juice, and cider vinegar.
Normal scalp: Softening ingredients like jojoba and aloe.

mane class

When it comes to hair care, think seasonally. During the winter, there's no humidity in the air, so hair flattens out as it loses moisture. Switch to lighter products and nongreasy formulas. For summer's high humidity, go with formulas that slick hair down and maintain shape and shine.

Problem: Frizzy

Try moisturizing shampoo and conditioner—avoid those containing protein, which can be drying. For curly hair, work antifrizz gel through hair and blow-dry using a diffuser attachment. For straight hair, apply straightening cream, then divide hair into sections. Using a big round brush to hold hair taut, blow-dry each section, aiming air down the hair shaft.

Fast fix: Finger-dry roots to avoid overheating. Use a lightweight detangling spray. Rub finishing emulsion between your palms and smooth over any frizz.

Problem: Greasy

For greasy hair that needs frequent washing, avoid using shine-enhancing products, which can make greasy hair look stringy. Don't use creamy conditioners and waxes that stay on the hair shaft and put your oil production into overdrive. Don't overbrush. Use a dab of leave-in conditioner on the ends only, avoiding the scalp.

Fast fix: Blot your scalp with oil-absorbing sheets intended for your face.

Problem: Lanky

Shampoo with a volumizing product, then apply a light conditioner to the ends. When your hair is 60 percent dry, apply five to ten spritzes of body-boosting spray to your roots. While blow-drying, lift sections of your hair with fingers or a vent brush and aim heat at the roots.

Fast fix: Lift your hair at the roots and spritz with light, flexible-hold spray.

Problem: Fly-away

Static electricity is caused by friction between your comb and your hair, and between individual hairs. Don't comb too often. Conditioners coat the hair, which provides insulation. Use the highest-level conditioner you can that doesn't weigh your hair down.

Fast fix: Lightly spray on leave-in conditioner or apply a few drops of silicone serum.

Problem: Hat head

A common sight in good weather when hats are worn to protect the hair from damaging UV rays, or in cold temperatures.

Fast fix: Blow-dry hair from roots to the end to add lift. Carry emergency tools along to fix hair later, like a barrette or clip.

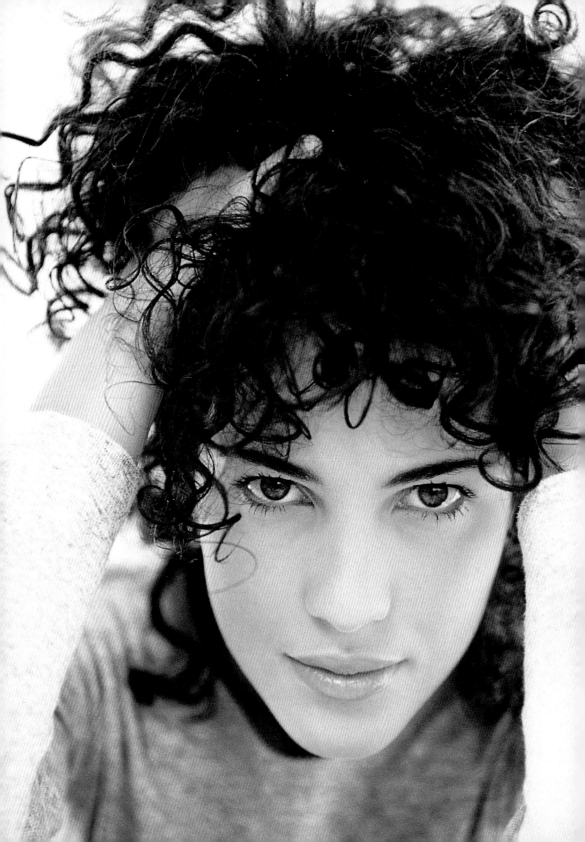

MANAGING IT

MANAGING IT

Half the battle is learning how to work with the head of hair you've been given. You may know best how your hair behaves, what it responds to, and what pitfalls to avoid, but getting hair to look healthy, shiny, and manageable can take a little knowledge, a lot of practice, and some firsthand expert advice.

The best haircuts are easy to style on your own and versatile so you can get a lot of looks out of them. It all starts at the salon. Sometimes it is hard to take a step back and figure out your hair options for yourself. A good stylist can look at you objectively and tell right away what will work for you and what won't.

No matter what kind of hair you have, every woman can have a bad hair day once in a while. There are days when you just can't be bothered or don't have the extra time it takes to devote to your style. Make a contingency plan. Your stylist can teach you the tricks you need to throw together a great look, no matter what mood you're in. Learning how to tie hair back, pile it up, or twist it around can be a lifesaver when you're pressed for time or not in the mood. For special occasions, a quick blow-dry by a professional is well worth the extra expense. No one can make your hair look as gorgeous and glam as an extra pair of talented hands.

scissor hands

One of the simplest ways to keep hair in peak condition is with frequent trims. Whether long or short, hair should be trimmed regularly, approximately every six to eight weeks.

Waiting longer between cuts allows ends to go dull and become susceptible to breakage. There is no miracle product to repair split ends. However much you are tempted, ignore the gimmicks. The only way to get rid of ends is to cut them off. When growing out layers, make sure you have a reshape on a regular basis. As well as keeping your hair healthy, this maintains maximum fullness.

TOP TIP:
Don't skimp. One of the best beauty investments you can make is to get a great hairdresser.

Hairstylists are usually the first people to notice any problems such as hair loss. They have the advantage of being able to see the back of your head without the awkwardness of holding a hand mirror. It is worth taking the time to find a hairdresser you bond with and who will be honest if there is a problem.

If you are trying to grow out layers or bangs, you will need frequent visits to the salon to maintain a style. When your next hair appointment is still two weeks away, the boldest souls may be tempted to start clipping. Unless you're desperate, don't trim your hair yourself. Most professional hairstylists will allow you to pop in to have your bangs touched up in between haircuts to keep your style in check.

If you have no option but to do it yourself, follow these tips to get the job done right. Use a straight comb with wide teeth, very sharp haircutting scissors (not the ones in your kitchen drawer), and gel to give you added control. Secure the rest of your hair, leaving only the bangs hanging loose to avoid any nasty accidents. Soft, wispy bangs that sweep along the eyebrows are the most flattering. They should frame your upper face and brow area. The endpoint should generally be your brow bone. Short, choppy bangs or those cut straight across can look more severe. Many women over forty enjoy the benefits of covering up forehead lines, wrinkles, and creases. Well-tailored bangs can camouflage an aging forehead or hairline that is too high. It can also save you a fortune in Botox shots.

Tearing your hair out

Ponytails and tight braids tug on hair and cause breakage. Always make ponytails using covered hair bands rather than the rubber ones you'll find in your desk drawer. Scrunchies, cloth-covered bands, and ribbons are a good alternative to thin elastic bands. The wider the band, the less tension on the hair. Vary where you place your ponytails from day to day, especially those placed high on the head, and give your hair a day off regularly to limit the stress on your hair. Be especially careful when you remove bands, clips, and barrettes from your hair because you can pull out hair that gets tangled in them. Choose hair clips that do not have sharp edges. Bungee elastics that have a hook at each end can be used to pull hair into a ponytail or bun without tangling hair, by wrapping them around your hair until it is tight enough and then just hooking the ends together.

the search for a stylist

Finding the right hairdresser is like dating—it's a long-term relationship and chemistry counts. Communication is also key. It may take time to get to know and understand each other.

- Ask for recommendations from friends. If you are out and about and see a woman with a hairstyle that you really like, ask her who she goes to.

- Go for a complementary consultation. Look around at the hairstylists and clients. Don't just put your head into someone's hands on a first visit.

- Get a list of prices for all the treatments offered to avoid a shock later. Choose a stylist you can afford to encourage more frequent visits.

- Tell your chosen stylist about your lifestyle, what you do for a living, and how much time you have to devote to your hair.

- Communicate the type of look and length you're going for and if you wear glasses, take them with you.

- If you don't like the way the cut is turning out, stop the hairstylist immediately to discuss it.

- If you think a different stylist in the same salon might suit you better, you can switch, even though it may feel awkward.

- One bad haircut doesn't mean you should switch stylists if you have been happy in the past.

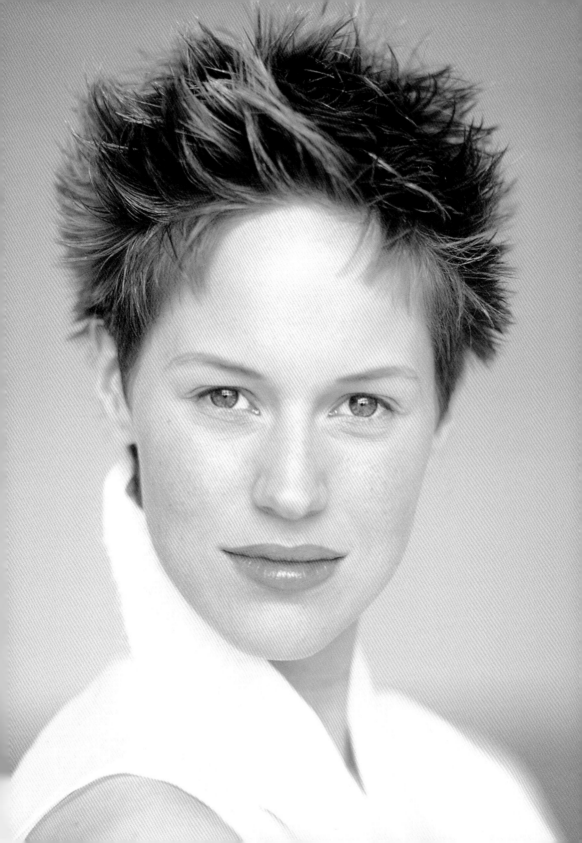

hot stuff

Of the many styling tools that use heat, the blow-dryer is the most commonly used. Curling irons come in second. Whatever you use, be careful not to damage your hair.

Nothing helps you achieve a fuller look than a blow-dryer in well-trained hands—it is an indispensable tool. However, the heat produced by styling tools can make chemical changes in hair, which in turn can cause discoloration and have a negative effect on the surface lipids and protein structure. Heat can literally boil out the water content in the hair shaft as it turns to steam, which severely damages the cortex. Overexposure to heat will make any type of hair look and feel dry and lifeless.

The heat is on

Approach blow-dryers with caution, especially if your hair is not in good condition to begin with. Always hold a blow-dryer at least six inches from your scalp and vary the temperature settings, using high heat only for short spurts. Keep the blow-dryer moving; don't hold it on one spot for too long. The hair concentration nozzle that comes with most blow-dryers helps keep hot coils as far away from the scalp as possible. The best ones to use have a narrow plastic nozzle with a thin slit that directs heat on one area at a time without ruining the adjacent section that you just finished drying. To dry hair like

BEAUTY BYTE:

For more tips on haircare, try www.behindthechair.com.

a pro, the rule is divide and conquer. Section off the front into thirds and secure each part with a clip. For thicker hair, make more sections. Diffusers—the cone-shaped attachments that fit on the barrels of blow-dryers—are good for diffusing the airflow over a larger area and drying hair more slowly. These work well for curly hair to hold the curl. The most effective blow-dryer should have enough power to get the job done—from 1,200–2,000 watts. Beware of cheaper models that often use more heat than needed.

The same rules apply when using curling irons. Go for one with a cool tip designed to use easily with one hand. Some models have an automatic safety shut-off switch to control the temperature settings. You can bake a cake at about 350°F, so imagine what your curling tongs are doing to your hair with their average temperature of 285°F. Blow-dryers are slightly cooler at 250°F, while hot rollers usually work at 212°F.

If you've been on an all-out blow-drying mission lately, your hair may feel like damaged goods. Give it a rest and time to repair itself. Try using a specially designed absorbent hair towel that can dry hair in record time. Towel drying can rough up the cuticle, which makes hair harder to comb through. Squeeze out excess water and wrap hair in a towel.

Some conditioning and styling products are heat-activated to get treatment directly to where the potential for damage is greatest. They can slow down keratin breakage and stimulate the metabolism of the hair root. Air-dry your hair naturally in the sun to avoid this type of damage.

frazzled follicles

frazzled follicles

Dry hair is a relative concept. Hair can react dramatically to the way you treat it. You may think your hair is dry because of insufficient moisture and oil content, but think again.

If your hair does not have a normal sheen or texture but is dry and brittle, it may be the result of excessive washing, harsh detergents, heat processing, or a dry or hostile environment. Friction is another culprit. Rough brushing or overcombing, even fabric pillows and pillowcases, can cause friction on the hair, which can be potentially damaging.

One way to combat the coarse, brittle look and texture of dry hair is by using conditioners. If your hair is on the dry side, use a conditioner after every shampoo to achieve softness and shine. Even conditioners cannot revitalize severely damaged hair. If your hair is constantly dry and intensive conditioning doesn't seem to help, see your doctor. Fragile hair that breaks easily may be a sign of more than just a problem of vanity. It may be caused by an underlying medical condition, such as metabolic diseases, hypothyroidism, or poor nutrition.

Abnormally dry, lifeless hair may also be a result of the natural oil being stripped from the cuticle due to any of a number of causes. Hair tends to dry out during the winter in cold climates and can become dry after the use of steam heat, long periods of sun exposure, or when a buildup of flakes clogs oil glands. Any tool that adds heat, like blow-dryers, curling irons, straightening irons, and electric rollers, can cause further damage to hair.

Directions: These should be used on clean hair that is partially dry or just damp, rather than on dripping wet hair when they weigh strands down. Avoid applying before using curling tongs, since the heat may cause your hair to stick to the tongs if the gel or mousse melts. Use a small dollop (the size of a quarter) squeezed into your palm. Rub palms together to spread evenly and apply lightly. Use mostly your fingertips to scrunch waves and curls, and an open palm to create a smoother, sleeker look. For longer hair, applying fixatives from midway down the hair will give a better hold. Comb through if needed to distribute evenly. Applying gels near the roots or brushing products through the hair will flatten out your curls.

Sprays: Styling sprays create your style, whereas holding sprays keep it in place. Stiff hairsprays are always a no-no. Avoid products labeled "maximum hold," which can defeat the purpose of adding volume to hair by making it sticky. Sprays that contain alcohol tend to be more drying; ditto for aerosols. Nonaerosols often provide less hold, but give a more natural look and feel. If your hair is thin or limp, use a fine misting spray. Holding sprays may contain polymers that act as the fixative. The finer the mist, the smaller the droplets deposited. Sprays also keep humidity out, which keeps your style in shape.
Directions: Spray a small amount evenly over your style from a distance of about one foot. Don't spritz too close to the hair, as this will cause buildup. You may want to reapply later in the day, so don't overuse.

Waxes and pomades: These should be reserved for thick, curly, and coarse hair types and should never be used on fine or limp hair. Waxes are heavier than pomades and work well to create spiky styles or tame unruly ends. Pomades are applied to slick hair down and keep it frizz-free in humid weather.
Directions: Use only a dab rubbed on the palms and/or fingertips to distribute evenly through the hair. Use sparingly to avoid a greasy, flat look.

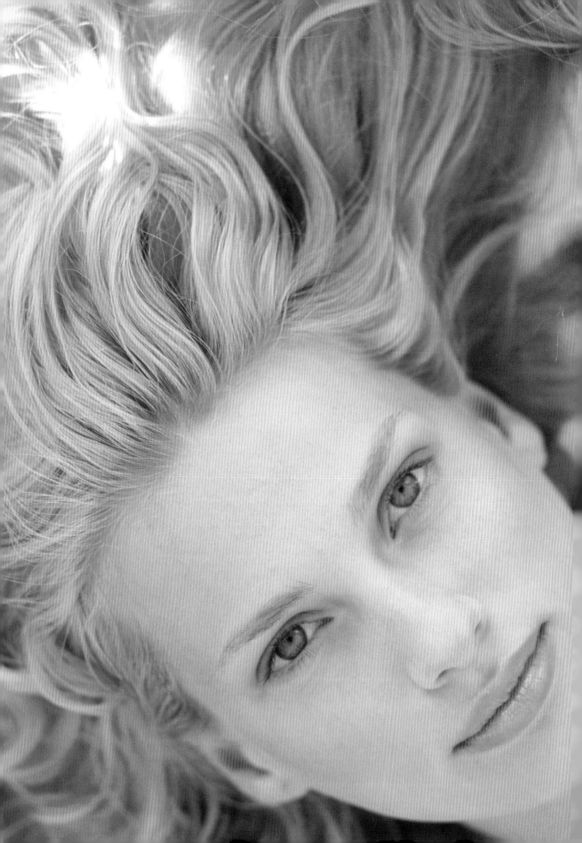

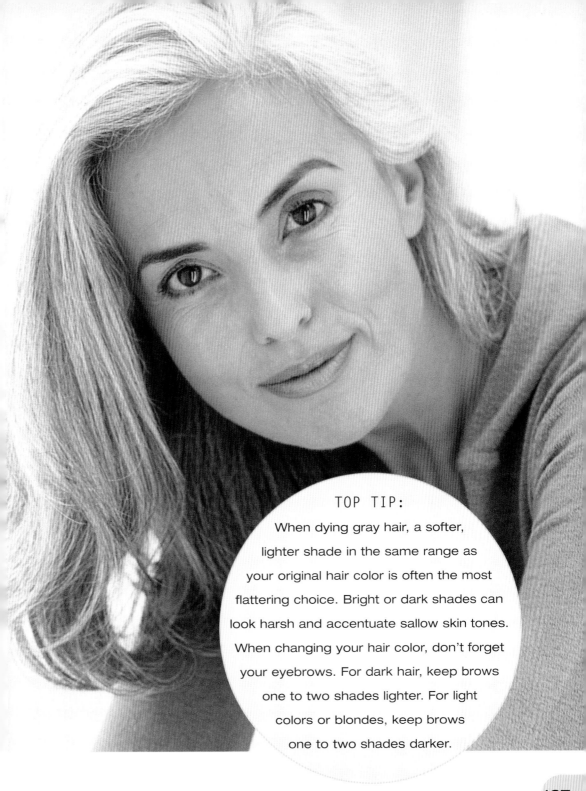

TOP TIP:

When dying gray hair, a softer, lighter shade in the same range as your original hair color is often the most flattering choice. Bright or dark shades can look harsh and accentuate sallow skin tones. When changing your hair color, don't forget your eyebrows. For dark hair, keep brows one to two shades lighter. For light colors or blondes, keep brows one to two shades darker.

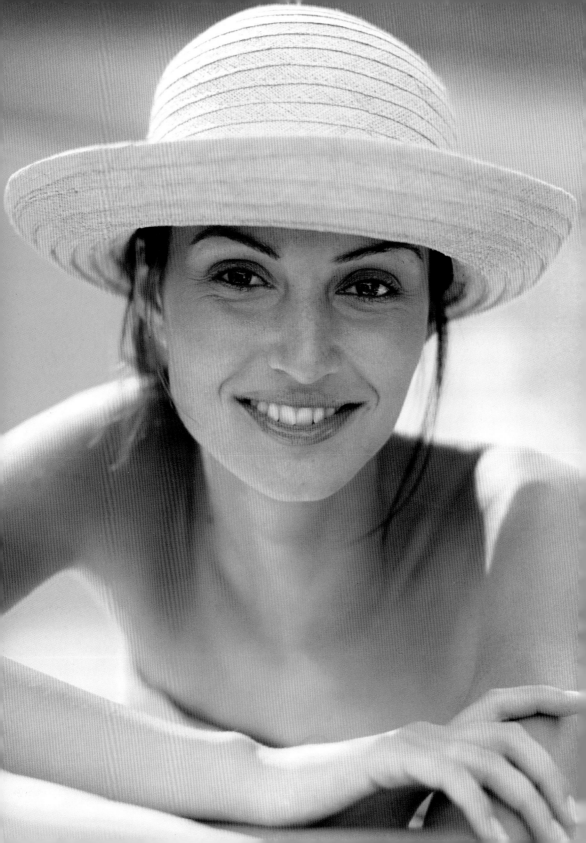

LOSING IT

LOSING IT

Being follically challenged is not a laughing matter. Hair loss is a natural part of the aging process, along with sagging necks, stained teeth, and wrinkles. Lost hair is often dismissed as another casualty on the road to getting older. While it can be the bane of your existence, thinning hair doesn't have to be the end of the world.

If you think you might be imagining a few extra hairs wedged between your bristles lately, you're not alone. Many women think thinning hair is a man's problem, but hair loss is more common in women than you think. For every five men with hereditary hair loss, there are three women with the same condition. It can begin as early as your twenties and is so common that, by the age of thirty-five, almost 40 percent of women demonstrate some of the signs. By fifty, half of all women will experience some degree of hair thinning.

Women often miss the early signs of thinning, thinking that their hair is simply becoming finer. Putting off seeking medical attention to find out why your hair is thinning can make the difference between effective treatment and having to live with it.

ages and stages

ages and stages

The life of the hair is similar to the life of the skin. In your twenties, you love your hair, then somewhere in your fourth decade, your first gray hair arrives. At first there are only a few and they are easy to pluck out, but with each passing decade, the number of gray hairs increases.

20s Hair grows fastest from the ages of sixteen to twenty-four • Strands turn darker • Oil glands work overtime

30s First stray gray hairs appear • Hair starts to get finer • Hair needs extra protection from damage

40s Gray hairs are coming in fast and furious • There are now too many gray strays to pluck • Due to a reduction in estrogen levels, hair thins and becomes drier and duller

50s The menopause and loss of estrogen contribute to further hair loss • Your long hair days are over • Hormone fluctuations can make you lose hair from the top of your head and grow it on your face

60s Your hair has turned from gray to white • The oil glands have slowed down, making hair drier • Your hair continues to thin out

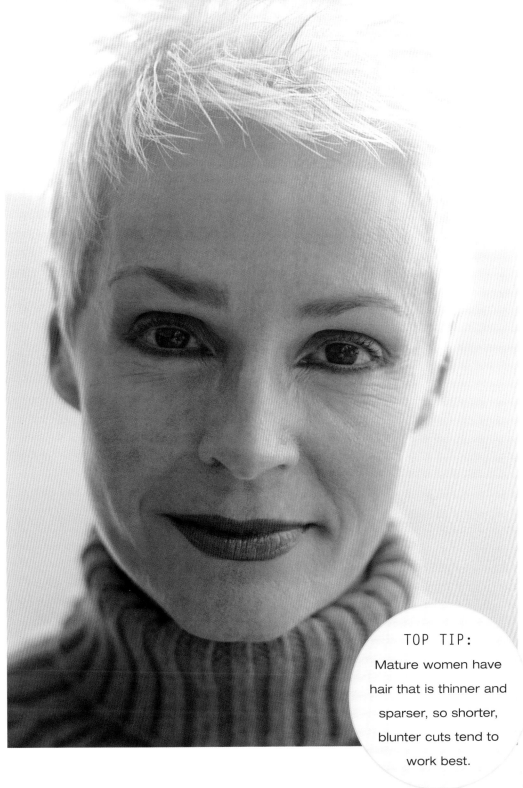

TOP TIP:
Mature women have
hair that is thinner and
sparser, so shorter,
blunter cuts tend to
work best.

thinning out of control

Hair is alive; it grows, it rests, it breaks, it dies, and unfortunately it falls out. It sometime grows back the same, less, or not at all.

The best way to keep it from falling out prematurely is to thicken what you've got from the inside out and to maintain its strength and condition. Finding hairs in your sink is not necessarily a sign of thinning hair; it could be going through the usual process or it could indicate a temporary hair loss condition. If you are not on your way to balding, your hair will grow back just as strong. If you are, however, your hair will grow back finer and will not grow as long as it used to before falling out again. If the cause is largely genetic, topical medications may be a good place to start. More serious hair-loss conditions require transplantation to help you keep up appearances.

If you are suffering from excessive hair loss, before you set off on a search for wigs or hair transplants, your first step should be a consultation with a dermatologist to determine the cause. The best time to begin treatment is in the early stages, when you first begin to display signs of hair loss. As with any medical condition, hair loss responds better to treatment if caught early.

Rooting out the cause is key

Female hair loss can be difficult to diagnose, as different conditions have a similar appearance. Causes range from genetics, hormonal flux, poor circulation, stress, rapid weight loss, and certain medications.

> TOP TIP:
> Female pattern hair loss can begin in the late teens to twenties, and can progress if left untreated.

The doctor will take a detailed medical history and possibly perform diagnostic tests to determine the cause of your hair loss. There are some health conditions that can go undetected, which contribute to hair loss. For example, an underactive or overactive thyroid gland and iron deficiency can make you shed too much hair. You may not know you have either condition and hair loss may be the first sign.

Diagnostic tests

Thyroid function tests: Checking the thyroid-stimulating hormone to rule out thyroid abnormalities.

Blood tests: Studies to measure blood lipids, complete blood count (CBC).

Hormone levels: DHEAS, testosterone, androstenedione, prolactin, follicular stimulating hormone, leutinizing hormone, to identify hormonal conditions.

Iron deficiencies: Serum iron, serum ferritin, total iron binding capacity (TIBC), to rule out anemia.

Venereal Disease Research Laboratory Test (VDRL): A test to rule out syphilis, a disease that can cause patchy hair loss.

After carefully examining the scalp and hair, further tests may be needed to zero in on the causes. These tests are used as a screening mechanism to determine general health, as well as specific abnormalities that may contribute to hair thinning. Once the underlying cause is identified—if one can be pinpointed—it should be treated. For example, if you have a thyroid condition, thyroid-replacement hormones may be prescribed. Women with heavy menstrual periods can develop an iron deficiency due to blood loss. If you have low serum iron, iron pills may be recommended.

getting the shaft

There are many reasons why your hair may be falling out, for starters, genetics, stress, diet, hormones, and chemicals. Some of these are entirely out of your control.

The most common cause of thinning hair is heredity and can be passed down from either your mother's or your father's side of the family. The more bald people there are in your family, the greater your chances of losing your hair. Contrary to common myth, it does not skip a generation. The propensity is passed down from any and all of your relatives. About half the people who have one balding parent of either sex will inherit the dominant gene for baldness.

FOLLICLE FACT:
Balding is predominant among Caucasians and more common in those with fine hair.

Hormonal flux

Periods of hormonal change are a common cause of female hair loss. Many women do not realize that they can lose their hair after pregnancy, following discontinuation of birth control pills, or during menopause. The changes that occur during pregnancy usually slow down the shedding process, which is why some women's hair becomes so nice and thick. Within a few months of childbirth, though, the hair that did not get shed during pregnancy sometimes seems to fall out all at once. Hair loss may not show up for three months following the hormonal change and it may take another three months for the normal growth pattern to fully resume.

Tress stress

Surgery, severe illness, and emotional stress can also have a negative impact on your hair. The body can simply shut down the production of hair during periods of stress, since it is not necessary for survival and instead devotes its energies toward repairing vital body structures. In many cases there is a three-month delay between the onset of stress and the first signs of hair loss. Furthermore, there may be another three-month delay before the return of noticeable hair regrowth. Thus, the total hair loss and regrowth cycle can last six months or possibly longer when caused by physical or emotional stress. Although they will not cause balding on their own, physical and emotional stress can adversely affect the quality and strength of the hair. Stress does not cause permanent hair loss.

Cosmetic surgery

One of the most common complaints women have after a facelift is that they are losing their hair, specifically along the sides of the head. Hair loss can also come as an unwanted surprise after a brow lift. The cause is often the tension of the suture or stitches placed in the hair follicles. Newer, more modified facelifts can be designed to avoid making any incisions in the hairline for this reason. The good news is that it's usually a temporary condition and regrowth occurs within the first three to four months. If you are already experiencing thinning hair and are contemplating a lift, talk to your surgeon to determine your risk level. Some plastic surgeons may recommend a twice-daily, four-month course of Minoxidil (see page 182) before and after surgery as a precaution.

diet details

Abnormal hair texture, sheen, and color may be a symptom of certain stages of malnutrition. Hair loss can be caused by fad dieting, eating disorders, or just not eating well.

Crash diets by their very nature don't meet the minimum Required Daily Allowance (RDA) levels. Temporary hair loss may occur as a result of the stress and shock that crash dieting can put on your internal systems. Protein or iron deficiencies may affect your hair count. From a dermatologist's standpoint, supplemental vitamin pills cannot prevent the hair loss that is associated with losing weight rapidly. Many over-the-counter diet supplements are high in Vitamin A, which can often make hair loss worse.

The simplest advice is to get sufficient vitamins and minerals in your diet by eating enough protein—meat, poultry, and soy—and foods containing essential fatty acids, especially olive oil and fish. Drinking three glasses of skim milk per day also helps. If you have difficulty getting enough essential nutrients into your diet, eat as healthily as you can and take a multivitamin supplement.

Treatments and supplements made from herbs and roots have been cited as cures for hair loss, but data is sketchy and there are no guidelines regarding correct dosage or side effects. Many studies have been done in countries where testing parameters are lax. None are scientifically proved to actually stop hair loss or encourage regrowth. Ask your doctor before taking anything.

BEAUTY BYTE:
To learn about hair loss in women, log on to www.womenshairinstitute.com.

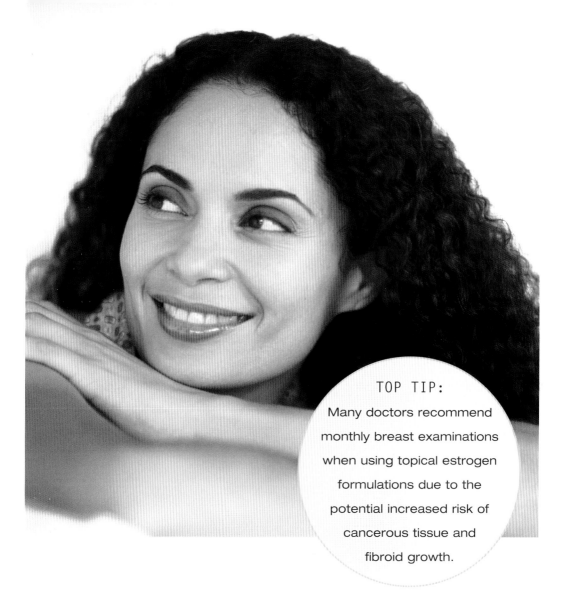

TOP TIP:

Many doctors recommend monthly breast examinations when using topical estrogen formulations due to the potential increased risk of cancerous tissue and fibroid growth.

to treat acne, overactive oil glands, and hirsutism. Studies have shown that saw palmetto may act in a similar way as an antiandrogen, although it has yet to be proven as a treatment for hair loss.

Expert advice: Experts agree that making dietary changes and using topical solutions offer the best combination treatment available, short of surgery.

fuzz buzz

Although there is an abundance of so-called remedies for baldness in a bottle, the only true way to restore your hairline is to get help from a specialist.

Hair transplantation, formerly one of the most tedious and labor-intensive cosmetic surgery procedures, is now a simple day surgery done under local anesthetic. The best type of procedure depends on the extent and pattern of hair loss. Often a combination of techniques will be needed. The ideal candidate for hair transplants is a woman who has either female-pattern or male-pattern baldness and enough hair on the back of the head to redistribute to where it is thinning. Female pattern baldness is progressive; the results you get today may not stay that way, so your surgeon has to plan your hairline and the density of transplanted hair for the long term.

Women are considered more challenging to treat for hair loss than men. As in most things, our expectations are higher. In a man, if he sees he has a little more on top and maybe looks a few years younger, he's usually satisfied. Women want thick, glossy hair all the time. Hair transplants can actually be simpler for women because they're able to hide them better. Women can easily wear scarves, and because women's hair is generally longer, it's harder to see the incision. When new hair begins to grow, the effect on a woman's scalp is more subtle. People may notice that your hair looks better but they won't be quite sure why. Something else to be aware of is that transplanting hairs next to existing hairs can bring on traumatic shock, which causes existing hairs to shed. This can lead you to actually look worse after a procedure than before. The shock loss is usually temporary, but since the existing hairs may also be damaged by pattern loss, it is possible they won't grow back. If the transplant is done carefully, so as not to disturb the existing hairs, it won't induce shock loss.

Hair transplants can be likened to planting cuttings. The technique moves your own hair follicles from the back or side of the head and transplants them to the thinning or balding areas, where they will regrow naturally. Done well, it can look very natural. After all, it's your own naturally growing hair. Small donor strips of hair-bearing scalp are removed from the back and sides of the head, which is an area of the densest hair for even the baldest heads. The area that grafts are taken from is called the "donor site." The beauty of the methods used today is that only ONE fine white scar in the back of the scalp is necessary. The surgeon can keep using the same hidden scar over and over for any transplant procedures that may be needed in the future. The strips of scalp are divided into grafts for placement in the balding areas. The hair-bearing grafts are carefully inserted into small holes or slits that are made in the balding scalp. The grafts can also be inserted between existing hairs to increase the density and thicken the area. Strategic planning and precise placement of grafts is essential to give the illusion of more hair.

REALITY CHECK: Approximately one third of women with thinning hair are candidates for hair transplants.

mini- & micrografts

Mini- and micrografts are the most commonly performed hair procedures for women, and they remain the treatment of choice.

The characteristics of your hair and scalp—including color, texture, skin-to-scalp contrast, curl, hair density, estimated future hair loss, and how much donor hair you have—determine whether you are a good candidate for a graft. Over the last decade, the basic size of hair grafts has become smaller and finer. Micrografts as small as single hairs are commonly placed behind the hairline to provide a gradually increasing density. They are ideal to fill in the hairline region, a common problem area for women. Most surgeons use a combination of variable-size grafts for the most natural-looking results.

Micrograft: One to two hairs into needle holes.

Small slit grafts: Three to four hairs into a slit recipient site.

Large slit grafts: Five to seven hairs into a slit recipient site.

Small minigraft: Three to four hairs into a small recipient site.

Large minigraft: Five to eight hairs into a small round recipient site.

A typical session takes two to three hours. It is now possible to move about 400–500 skin grafts—of two to four hairs each—from the back of the head to the front and top in one session. Initially the donor hair falls out within a few weeks or months, but regrows about three months later. Within four to six months, you can see a huge difference, and it continues to grow for as long as the hair would have done had it been left in the site from which

BEAUTY BYTES:

For more information, log on to www.ahlc.org, hairtransplants.com, and www.ishrs.org.

it was removed. Despite improvements, transplants are labor intensive and require the skill of a surgeon along with a team of three to five assistants. Megasessions can deliver 3,000–4,000 grafts, taking ten to twelve hours and involving several technicians. The amount of density that you can achieve depends on the number of grafts placed per session. Most women only require one or two treatment sessions for a good correction.

Lasers

The holes or slits needed to reposition hair follicles can be made with the aid of Erbium:YAG or carbon dioxide laser technology. The laser creates very small punctures of a consistent depth and width, which in some cases can speed up the length of time the procedure takes. It causes less bleeding and incurs a shorter healing time than was previously necessary.

Future shock

Recombinant DNA gene therapy is the most likely prospect as a cure for baldness. Researchers have pinpointed the first human gene linked to baldness, which may provide key information on how hair grows. Through gene therapy, it may be possible to give you back the gene that codes you for a particular deficiency. Creams that contain the gene may eventually be developed, meaning it can be transferred via the body into the bloodstream. Alternatively, topical creams could be applied directly to the hair follicle.

Scientists are currently working on hair cloning—a tissue-engineering technique that uses a single hair follicle to create thousands more, which can then be inserted into a bald area of the scalp. The technology already exists. Growing new hair follicles from existing ones could actually increase the number of hairs on your head, instead of just repositioning them as conventional hair replacements do.

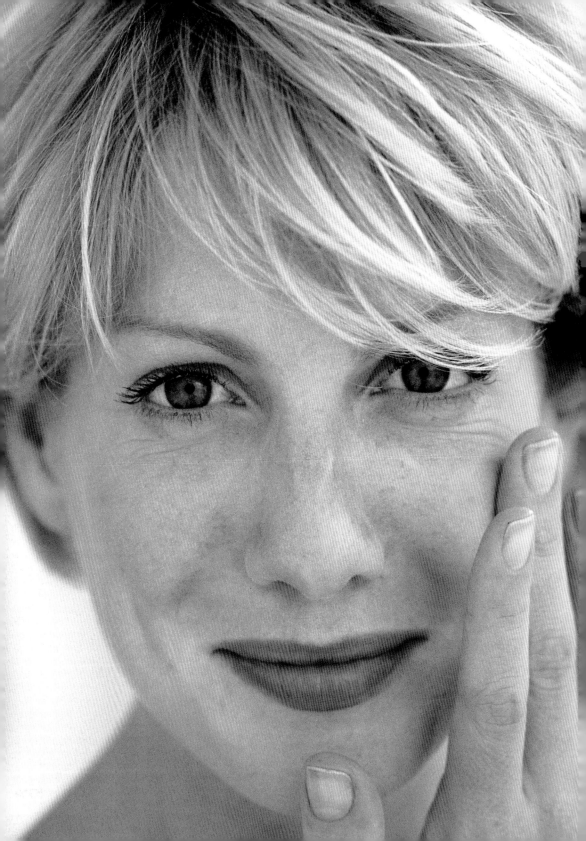

WRINKLE RESCUE

WRINKLE RESCUE

Our life expectancy has reached an all-time high. Women born in 1970 can expect to live an average of almost eighty years. The sad fact is that we all age, but looking older is a matter of choice. With modern technology, you can hold off looking old for longer.

Wrinkles form largely because levels of collagen—a component of the connective tissue in the skin that creates flexibility—decrease over time. There are two major ways that skin ages: intrinsic aging, which is genetically programmed and affects the skin all over your body; and photoaging, resulting from the long-term effects of sun, smoking, and pollution. The degree to which skin photoages is also determined genetically to some extent. Fair-skinned people tend to photoage more and earlier than those with dark skin.

The earlier you start caring for your complexion, the better it will serve you over the long haul. Antiwrinkle treatments can undo damage, but prevention is best. Eighty percent of the lines and wrinkles you see in the mirror were caused by the sun. The other 20 percent result from smiling, pouting, and frowning. If you have not paid your skin its due respect, all is not lost. It is never too late to start preventing new wrinkles, or to begin therapy to soften the ones you have.

face facts

The skin that gets exposed to those nasty UV rays the most—your face, neck, and hands—will age fastest.

Similarly, skin that is the thinnest on the body—the delicate eyelid area—is most susceptible to damage, lines, and aging. The skin is the body's first defense against disease and infection. It is the body's largest organ, protecting internal organs from injury. It regulates body temperature, prevents excess fluid loss, and helps remove any water and salt the body doesn't need. It also protects against light, infection, and environmental elements.

Thinning skin is a result of a breakdown of collagen fibers. Skin loses elasticity, especially if it has been exposed to excessive sunlight and becomes fragile. Skin dries out because the structure weakens and it doesn't retain moisture as well as younger skin. With menopause comes declining estrogen levels. Skin usually gets drier, however some women become oilier even if they never had oily skin as a teenager. The skin may also be affected by diuretics and certain medications, such as those for blood pressure.

Dry skin may suggest that your skin is lacking the nutrients it needs to stay healthy. Topical agents such as wrinkle creams and moisturizers help give the top layer of skin the vitamins and minerals that can help this layer look younger and healthier. Not every face needs a moisturizer and of those that do, not all require daily applications. If your skin is dry, moisturize it. The drier it is, the heavier the moisturizer you need. If your skin is naturally oily, there is no need to add extra moisture to it. The amount of natural lubrication or sebum produced by the skin declines with age.

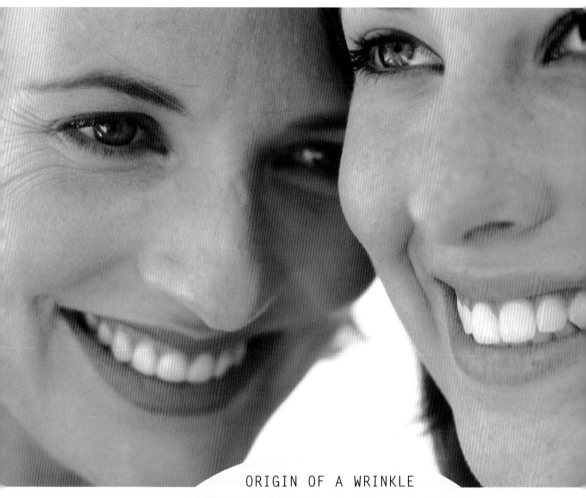

ORIGIN OF A WRINKLE

Fine wrinkles: Caused by the breakdown of collagen and elastin fibers over time.

Deep wrinkles: Caused by the building up of muscle in the deep layers below the surface of the skin.

Dynamic wrinkles: Only visible when muscles are engaged, as in smiling or frowning.

Static wrinkles: Seen all the time, when the face is at rest or moving.

skin aging

So you think your skin is going to look young forever. Guess again! At thirty, it takes on a life of its own. Your mission is to outsmart your skin cells before they get the better of you.

20s **Skin heaven:** Your skin is clear of blemishes, your pores are invisible, and your complexion is even and taut. Save your skin by using an SPF 15 every day and getting your tan out of a bottle, tube, or spray. Start your preventive antiaging regime with a good eye cream to hold off crow's-feet. Cleanse well, remove all traces of dirt and makeup before going to bed, and keep oil plugs at bay with good exfoliation.

30s **Party's over:** Expect to see visible changes in your skin's texture. This can be a real eye-opener. Cell turnover gently slows down, so adding exfoliants to speed it up is key. It's the perfect time to start more intense antiaging skin care. Collagen and elastin fibers begin to break down, so keep them firm by integrating nutrients into your program like Vitamin C, AHAs, antioxidants, and plant enzymes. Smokers will start to see fine lines around the mouth and squinters will spy their first crow's-feet. It's the ideal time to get professional advice about treatments like Botox, peeling treatments, and lasers for spider veins.

40s   **They're here:** Your wrinkles are in full force, so it's time to bring out the heavy artillery. Everything becomes lazy: Skin gets drier, and sagging and wrinkles give way to folds, furrows, and creases. Your brow droops and the corners of your mouth turn down as jowls creep up. The best plan is to fight back with medically advanced skin-care formulas that are worth spending money on. Look for high-tech ingredients like antioxidants and enzymes, which should keep your face and neck supple. Wage war on brown spots with lightening agents. Stick to a regime of facial peels, Botox, and wrinkle fillers to combat creases. This is the time to start investigating surgical options to plan for your beauty future.

50s   **Desperate measures:** It's a big number, but don't let it get you down. Turn back the clock with rejuvenating treatments, moisturizing serums, and firming masks. Your hormones are wreaking havoc, accounting for enlarged pores and increased oil activity. At this stage, you will get limited results from para-surgical treatments. Once your jawline starts to soften and the nasal labial folds require lots of filling, the time has come to nip or tuck. Facelift techniques have come a long way. With shorter scars and faster healing, they are the mainstay in a woman's arsenal against aging. By having your first lift before you turn fifty, you may never have to go public. It won't make you look twenty again, but it can keep your big birthday a secret for longer.

skin care jungle

Examine your face and let that be your guide. Your skin looks different every day, so adjust your skin care accordingly. Add, delete, or substitute products and treatments as needed.

The factors that determine how long your skin will stay glowing include genetics, diet and nutrition, sun exposure, whether you smoke or drink heavily, and stress levels. The best defense you've got is to protect your skin from free-radical damage and make use of therapies that go on a search-and-destroy mission to neutralize these little molecules. Repairing skin that has visible signs of aging will not happen overnight. It is like starting an exercise program—start slow, gradually increasing your tolerance in stages. As with exercise, if you stop, the problem comes back again. Every woman is constantly looking for the perfect skin-care regime; a cleanser that removes makeup and leaves skin feeling comfortable, a toner that refreshes without drying, and a moisturizer that hydrates without clogging pores. A great skin-care regime involves more than one product and varies from one face to another.

Hot water and soap dissolve the skin's natural moisture, so keep your daily shower short and water temperature moderate. While bathing, rub your body with a washcloth to exfoliate. Gently pat yourself dry. If you rub too hard at either point, you may remove too much skin and contribute to further dehydration. While the skin is still damp, apply a moisturizer. In general, the heavier the moisturizer, the better it works on dry skin. When the skin becomes dry, it needs water to help rejuvenate it, and moisturizers trap water in the skin. Relief for dry skin typically comes in these forms: ointments, creams, oils, and lotions.

Ointments are thick, greasy, and best for preventing moisture from escaping from the skin. These are inconvenient for regular use. Ointments are best saved for areas that take a lot of abuse, such as hands, elbows, and feet. Creams are heavier than lotions and more effective at sealing in moisture for normal to dry skin. Oils are easily absorbed when applied to slightly damp skin after you pat dry, but often less moisturizing than ointments, creams, or lotions. Lotions are thinner and lighter so are least effective at replacing lost moisture in very dry skin. They evaporate quickly, making them the most convenient to use. They are often preferred over ointments and creams because they apply and absorb more easily. They are good for normal, oily, and young skin types that don't need as much added hydration. Lotions are also generally good for the body, but are less effective at sealing moisture in than ointments or creams. Eye creams are specially formulated for delicate eyelid skin. Some face and neck formulas will be too heavy around the eyes. If your eyes are puffy, use a lighter formula. Thicker ones will trap too much moisture in the skin and cause swelling.

Cleanse (and tone): Use a basic, gentle, nondetergent cleanser and make sure to rinse off all residue. You only need to use a toner if your skin doesn't feel clean without it, you are in a humid atmosphere, or you have oily or acne-prone skin.

Exfoliate: All skins need some form of exfoliation, but the degree will differ.

Treat: This phase encompasses everything from treating acne and eczema and bleaching dark spots to oil control and antiaging.

Moisturize: Skin needs hydration, but not all skin needs the same amount. Oily skin needs less and may not need any in particularly pimple-prone areas. The eyelid area needs more because it has the fewest oil glands.

Protect: Every skin needs UVA/UVB protection daily with a minimum SPF 15, all year long.

> TOP TIP:
> A quick-fix approach to skin care is destined to fail. Take the time to get educated and don't be afraid to ask for help when you need it.

PREVENTING THEM

PREVENTING
THEM

An ounce of prevention is worth a pound of cure in future wrinkle remedies. The best way to deal with wrinkles is not to get them in the first place. Protecting the skin from the sun is the single most important practice in skin care. Continuous sun exposure will wrinkle and dry out the skin, leaving it coarse and thick. Uneven pigmentation, freckles, and dark patches are also side effects. The earliest warning sign of severe skin damage is the development of actinic keratoses. These precancerous lesions are most common in people with fair skin and light hair, but can affect any skin type.

As you get older, your cumulative sun damage will start to crop up when you least suspect it. The sun's rays are very unforgiving, and the damage they do to the skin is inescapable. Products used for prevention don't necessarily produce visible results. For example, your sunscreen won't reduce wrinkles, but consistent use will keep them from forming as quickly and as deeply.

The first step in a program to revise the signs of aging should be the introduction of the new generation of "cosmeceuticals," which, by definition, are cosmetics that exert a pharmacologic effect on the skin.

ray bans

Approximately 5 percent of the UV radiation hitting the skin is reflected. The remaining 95 percent passes into the tissue, gets scattered, then passes out again or gets absorbed by molecules in the various layers of the epidermis and dermis.

UVA rays are longer than UVB rays, so they can penetrate more deeply through the skin's surface, where they kill collagen and elastin, which makes your skin slack and causes dry, leathery, blotchy patches. How wrinkled your skin gets depends largely on how much sun you have been exposed to in your lifetime. People who spend a lot of time outside without adequate protection develop leathery skin earlier, which makes them look older than they are.

Light spectrum

The longer the wavelength, the greater the energy level and the more damage it can do.

UVA are longer wavelengths, mostly transmitted to the dermis to be absorbed by hemoglobin in the blood or reflected back up and out of the body, but known to cause damage in the deep skin layers, as well as skin cancer.

UVB are shorter wavelengths, largely removed in the epidermis, particularly by DNA and melanin, and known to cause sunburn and skin cancer.

When it comes to your complexion, free radicals make the difference between "peaches 'n' cream" and "wrinkled prune." UV radiation has many effects on the skin as a result of its absorption by skin molecules, called chromophores, the most important of which is DNA. After UV absorption, DNA undergoes chemical changes. If these alterations are not repaired, they can be highly disruptive to the way cells function. It is now known that even small amounts of sunlight on the skin can cause DNA damage throughout the entire thickness of the epidermis. Fortunately, most of this is repaired within days, although some permanent damage may remain. The absorption of UV radiation by skin chromophores and the unrepaired damage are considered the main causes of visible skin damage. All levels of the skin are affected, but because UVB is largely absorbed high up before it reaches the dermis, most of the immediate damage is to the epidermis. UVA makes up approximately 95 percent of the ultraviolet light that we are exposed to.

When DNA is damaged by UVB exposure, chemicals are released that are important in repairing other skin molecular structures and which cause underlying blood vessels to swell. This is what shows up as sunburn. These chemicals may also contribute to harming the collagen and elastin fibers in the dermis, helping to speed up aging. If, after severe sunburn, the damage is so extensive that the cell cannot repair itself and dies, the skin blisters and peels.

REALITY CHECK:
Longer UVA and UVB wavelengths can pass through the atmosphere even on a cloudy day. They also penetrate car windows and sunglasses.

photoaging

To judge the effects of the sun on your skin, compare the appearance of areas that have not been exposed to the sun to your face, hands, and chest.

Those areas normally covered by clothing are smoother and tend to have fewer freckles and wrinkles. Facial skin, in contrast, may be freckled or dry and often looks dull, blotchy, and deeply wrinkled. It can also become covered with spider veins.

Photoaging is the result of accumulated skin damage caused by UV radiation over many years. As with sunburn, UVB wavelengths have the greatest impact. The potentially deeper-reaching UVA rays may affect you if you spend a lot of time on a sunbed or sunbathing, using a sunscreen that only blocks UVB rays. When the body is unable to fully repair damage to the DNA in the cells of the epidermis and the dermis, their structure deteriorates. Skin thickness increases with age, while skin elasticity decreases. Unfortunately, these changes cannot be avoided and can be irreversible. Sunlight also causes changes to the melanocytes, which gradually stop functioning so that your skin develops brown spots, blotchiness, or a yellowish hue. The epidermis becomes more fragile. All these changes combine to make up the visible signs of skin photoaging.

REALITY CHECK:
The only safe tan is a fake tan. Tanning parlors are Public Enemy #1 and a wrinkle's best friend.

Never too early to start

Start your sun protection program early, preferably while you're still in diapers. It has been estimated that up to 50 percent of your total UV radiation exposure is acquired by the age of eighteen, and 75 percent by the age of thirty.

If your photoaging clock has been ticking for some time, minimize further changes by being careful in the sun from now on. Photoaging steadily develops even if you are simply taking a walk around the block or sitting at a sidewalk café. The skin doesn't need to turn red, pink, or burn for slow, permanent damage to take place. Sunburn is a skin-repair process. Tanning is the release of UV-protective pigment following UV-induced DNA damage. Accumulated skin damage over many years produces deep wrinkles. Although the skin on your face may never look as young as the skin on your buttocks, it will look much better if you protect it from sun exposure. Practicing "safe sun" and avoiding tanning beds are a MUST.

SEVEN SIGNS OF PHOTOAGING

- Dehydrated and thickened outer skin layers
- Flaking and rough skin
- Age spots and sunburn freckles
- Sallow complexion
- Enlarged pores clogged with sebum
- Broken, enlarged capillaries
- Milia or small white cysts

The three key concepts are: prevention first, then maintenance, and when all else fails, correction. Making good decisions in skin rejuvenation isn't about loading up on every product out there or finding one that is better than all the rest. It's about incorporating at least two good ingredients that work in a complementary fashion and are appropriate for your skin type.

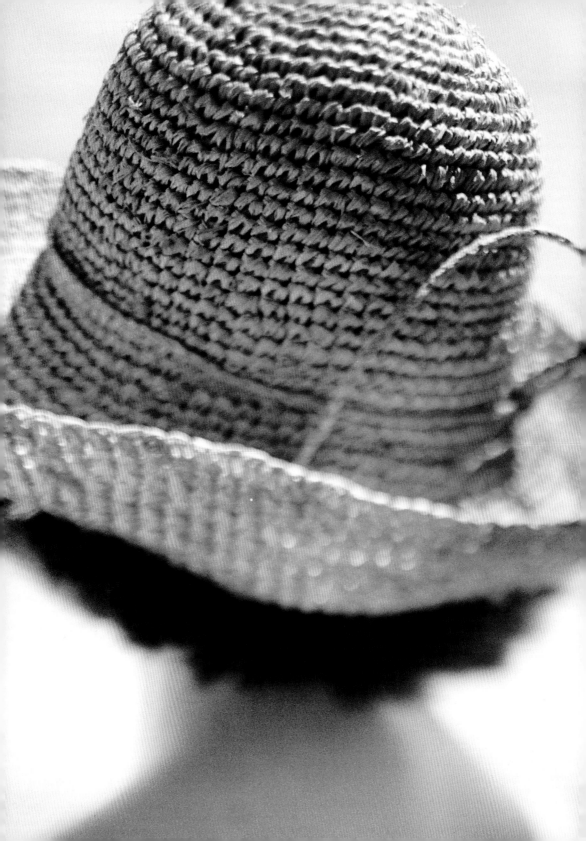

SPF savvy

Sunscreens temporarily absorb ultraviolet rays. The best formulas protect against both UVA—the culprit in wrinkle formation—and UVB, which causes tanning and burning.

The higher the Sun Protection Factor (SPF) rating, the stronger and longer its effects. The SPF index only addresses UVB rays. For protection against UVAs, look for products containing Parsol 1789, zinc oxide, or titanium dioxide.

> **TOP TIP:**
> When it comes to sunscreen, rub it on, rub it in well, rub it all over, and rub it on often.

The burning question is: "How much do I really need?" Sunblock should come in a six-pack, because most of us use far too little of it to be effective. Very few people use sunscreen every day, all year round. Fall and winter are no exception, no matter where you live or travel to.

Screen versus block

Sunscreen is a chemical agent that denatures light, making the wavelengths incapable of causing damage.

Sunblock is an agent that acts as a physical barrier to prevent sunlight from reaching the surface of the skin.

Some sunscreen formulas combine a mixture of the two concepts. More sensitive skin types may tolerate physical blockers better. Sunscreens with a heavier coating provide a better physical barrier.

screening room

Does your sun protection pass the test? With so many types on the market, it's hard to know which one is best for you.

Always use a minimum of SPF 15. Use SPF 30 for more intense exposure. Choose products that offer broad-spectrum protection (both UVA and UVB). For pimple-prone skin, use an oil-free or noncomedogenic sunscreen. Sunscreens with physical blockers, which lie on the skin's surface, are widely available. The new mineral sunscreens are lighter and wearable under makeup. Zinc oxide is the more potent and more expensive, so titanium dioxide is more widely used.

The difference in texture between cosmetic sunscreens for daily protection and sport sunscreens for outdoor and beach protection is waterproofing. Waterproof lotions have an oil base, which is thicker and heavier and can clog pores. When a product is labeled "water resistant," it should specify the length of time it will last if you come into contact with water. Labeling varies from country to country and there is still no standardization. Many dermatologists believe that over SPF 15, the differences in protection levels are very small, but SPF 15 is the minimum you need for it to be effective. Bump that up to SPF 30 if you are playing sports or are on a vacation where you are outdoors more than usual, skiing, swimming, or strolling.

Using a moisturizer that contains a sunscreen can also be misleading. You are unlikely to apply as much of it or use it as often as a regular sunscreen, so it will not be as effective. It may be adequate if you apply it all over your face and neck daily if your sun exposure is limited. It would not be considered enough protection for a day at the beach or playing tennis. What you use on your body is not the same as what you would choose for your face. Most women tend to buy two different sun products; one for the body and one with a higher SPF for the face. Choose a moderately priced formula for your body so you'll use more of it. It is critical that you like the feel, fragrance, and texture, to ensure that you use it daily. For your face, splurge on an elegant product that you enjoy using.

TOP TIP:

The best sun protectors are a wide-brimmed hat and protective clothing, especially the kind made with cool, light, tightly woven fabrics that keep the sun's rays out. Sunglasses with polarized lenses offer protection for your eyes and from crow's feet.

A fair blonde vacationing in the Caribbean generally needs more protection than an olive-skinned brunette walking down the street in March. The key is that whatever your sunscreen of choice, you must use enough of it and use it regularly. Dermatologists recommend using one ounce of lotion per application for one person's whole body.

Even if a foundation contains a sunscreen, facial movements throughout the day remove some of it from your face, decreasing its effectiveness. Foundations, concealers, moisturizers, eye creams, and lipsticks that offer UVA and UVB protection may be sufficient for normal daily activities. Sebum is produced during the day, thus separating the foundation from the skin's surface. Everyone experiences this, but normal to dry skin types will find it develops at a slower rate. When you are outside for a long period, your foundation will only protect you for about two hours. After that, either reapply foundation or use a sunscreen over it for continued protection.

TOP TIP:
Don't forget to cover the most burn-prone areas: your lips, eyelids, back of neck, tip of nose, forehead, chest, shoulders, and ears.

skin sins

If you want to defy aging, stop smoking and drink less alcohol. Nothing ages skin faster and dehydrates your pores mores than a cigarette and a glass of wine.

You can ALWAYS tell a smoker by her skin. It has a gray or sallow cast, feels dry, and is usually lined prematurely—early to mid-thirties—especially around the mouth and eyes. Even if you only have a few cigarettes a day, expect the telltale wrinkles around the mouth and eyes to appear in your thirties.

Scientists have an explanation for what makes smokers look old before their time. Tobacco has been found to activate the genes responsible for the skin enzyme that breaks down collagen, the protein that maintains elasticity in the skin. When this starts to disintegrate, the skin begins to sag and wrinkle. Too much of the enzyme increases the aging effect of the sun's rays, which also raises the concentration of the enzyme.

Smokers are more prone to getting wrinkles and their skin tends to have a grayish pallor. Smoking causes a flood of free radicals to form in the body, which speeds up the aging process. Research suggests that smokers have lower levels of vitamin C in their blood than nonsmokers, and that their daily loss of vitamin C is about thirty-five milligrams a day greater than nonsmokers'. Women who smoke need to consume at least 110 milligrams a day of vitamin C to compensate for this loss.

The combination of smoking and sunlight is positively deadly. Plus, the nicotine stains on your teeth and fingers are far from

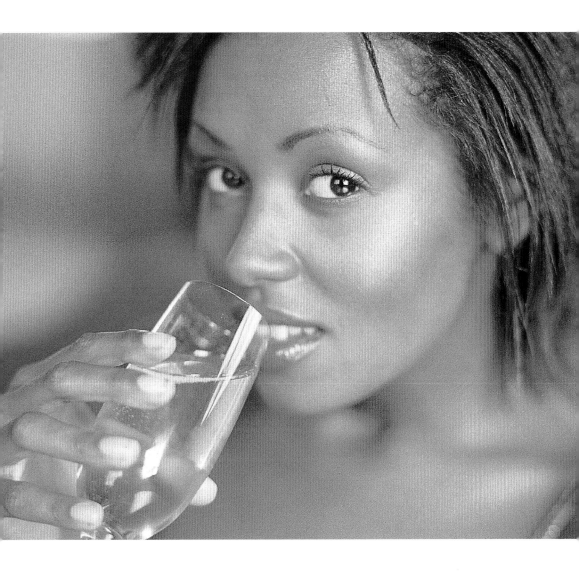

glamorous. The best beauty treatment, and the cheapest by far, is to
QUIT SMOKING.

Similarly, steer clear of overindulging on skin-aggravating alcohol.
Aside from hangovers, alcohol can wreak havoc on your skin and give
you a puffy face, red and irritated eyes, and a washed-out complexion.
Alcohol is a diuretic and causes blood vessels to dilate and the skin to
lose moisture, resulting in dehydration, sagging, and a loss of resiliency.
To help your skin stay wrinkle-free, keep cocktails to a minimum.

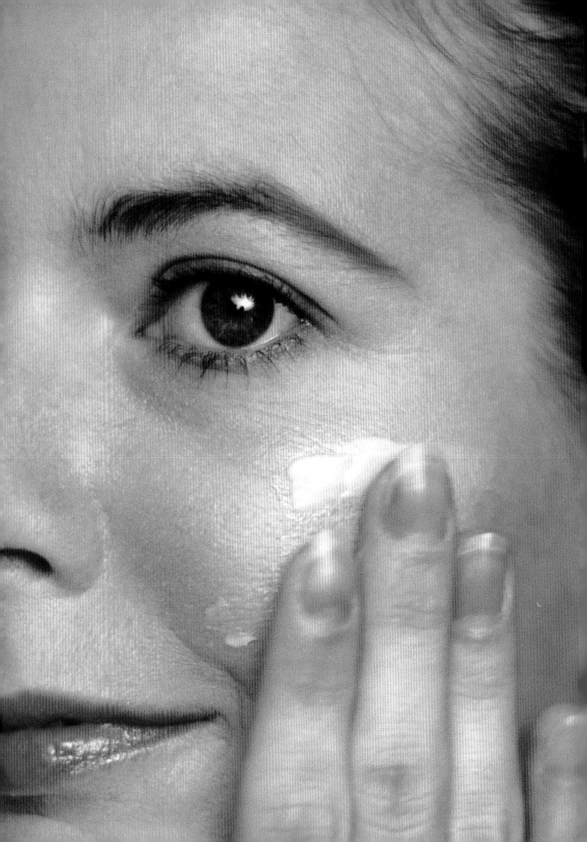

SMOOTHING THEM

SMOOTHING THEM

The aging process is under intense scrutiny by the scientific community. Every skin care product today has some combination of vitamins. The trick is to look for high concentrations of vitamins and antioxidants in stable enough forms to be applied topically. Retinoic acid, L-ascorbic acid, and alpha hydroxy acids have been the mainstays for aeons, but that's just the beginning. While they tackle skin aging in scientifically different ways, they work synergistically when used together.

Currently there are several clinically-proven active ingredients used in skin rejuvenation, plus a plethora of antioxidants and a vast array of ingredients that play a supporting role. Vitamin A, glycolic acid, N-6 Furfuryladenine, copper peptides, dimethylaminoethanol (DMAE), L-ascorbic acid, and alpha lipoic acid are the star performers.

Exfoliation means stripping away the old to bring in the new. On the skin this translates as radiance, vitality, and clarity. As cells clump together, you need to jump-start the natural process of sloughing off. There are many modern tools for exfoliation, from sponges, loofahs, and special washcloths and wipes, to peeling agents that penetrate the skin.

beauty boosters

If you're approaching thirty, consider adding a few "active" products to your skin care program to make sure you reap the benefits of today's advanced technologies.

The term "active" describes a product containing an ingredient that works beneath the skin's surface, producing visible changes. The active substance should appear in the first three to five ingredients on the list. For an ingredient to work, it has to be protected from air and light, reach the target tissue in an active form, be delivered in a high enough concentration to be effective, and be used on a regular basis.

Antiaging skin-care formulations fall into three classifications: over-the-counter (cosmetics); nonprescription (cosmeceuticals); prescription (drugs). Cosmeceuticals include bioactives that have antiaging, moisturizing, firming, and skin-lightening effects. The cosmeceutical category is considered the most scientifically reliable and potent because the products generally contain the highest concentrations of active ingredients.

Beauty and the lab

The key in this age of product overload is to read labels. New compounds are turning up in cleansers, moisturizers, and sunscreens all the time. It's hard to keep up, especially when some ingredients go by more than one name. By law, the first ingredient listed on the label should have the highest concentration in the formula, but every ingredient is listed, even when there are only trace amounts of it in the product.

Skin vitamins

Arnica: A botanical derived from a mountain plant, with antiseptic, astringent, antimicrobial, and anti-inflammatory properties.

Copper peptides: Known to aid in the healing of wounds.

Gluconolactone: One of the polyhydroxy acids that occurs naturally in the cells.

Hyaluronic acid: A polysaccharide naturally found in the body's connective tissues, used as a moisturizing agent in cosmetics.

Lactobionic acid: Contains gluconic acid, one of the polyhydroxy acids, found to aid in wound-healing and decreasing scaling.

L-ascorbic acid: Commonly known as vitamin C, a water-soluble antioxidant, known for its ability to destroy free radicals.

L-Glutathione: Found in all human tissues, a potent antioxidant amino acid that accelerates wound healing.

Linoleic acid: A liquid essential fatty acid that acts as a moisturizing agent.

Panthenol: Vitamin B5, a humectant that attracts water to the dermis to increase hydration.

Tea tree oil: A natural preservative with antiseptic and germicidal properties, also used in acne preparations.

Vitamin C Ester: A nonacidic, lipid-soluble antioxidant that delivers vitamin C to the skin.

Vitamin K: Used to lessen redness and reduce the appearance of broken capillaries and bruising.

acid test

AHAs are a group of acids, from fruits and other natural substances, that speed up cell turnover, improve texture, reduce fine lines, and even out skin tone.

AHAs are key to unclogging embedded cellular debris from pores and shedding the outermost layer of dead skin. They work by consistently peeling away dead and thickened areas of the skin, in essence thinning the buildup. If you stop using AHAs, your skin's turnover rate will gradually become more sluggish. With continued use, AHAs have been proven to improve a wide range of skin conditions including wrinkles, acne, blotches, and age spots. Other benefits include their moisturizing, oil reduction, and pore-cleansing abilities, as well as bleaching properties for lightening discoloration.

Over-the-counter AHA strengths vary from 4 to 15 percent, but are often neutralized to a degree that they are not very effective—8 percent is considered the baseline level needed to see results. You will only see visible improvement for as long as you are using the product. AHAs have the potential for irritation if you use the wrong strength or too much of the right one. Most skin types can use some form, but very sensitive skin types may only be able to tolerate the mildest, like polyhydroxy acids. Glycolic acid is thought to be the most effective AHA for skin rejuvenation because it helps draw other treatments deeper into the skin. At a low pH, it can also aid in stimulating collagen production within the dermis.

As the skin becomes conditioned to hydroxy acids, stronger concentrations can be used

WARNING: AHAs can irritate skin if the pH is too high or your skin is very sensitive. Start out with milder formulas under 8% or polyhydroxy acids.

Natural exfoliants

Glycolic acid: Most common AHA, derived from sugarcane or made from synthetic ingredients. Because it is a small molecule, it penetrates the skin easily.

Malic acid: Derived from apples and white grapes.

Tartaric acid: A type of glycolic acid that results from the fermentation process used in making wine.
Uses: Exfoliation, reducing surface oils, unclogging blackheads, smoothing fine lines.

Beta hydroxy acid: Also referred to as salicylic acid. It does not penetrate as deeply into the dermis as glycolic acid, so it is less irritating.
Uses: Exfoliation of epidermis, prevention of clogged pores.

Citric acid: Derived from citrus fruits. Acts as an antioxidant on the skin.
Uses: May stimulate collagen production, has mild bleaching properties.

Lactic acid: Comes from sour milk. Works as an exfoliator and to hold water in the skin as a component of the skin's natural moisturizing mechanism.
Uses: Softening thick, rough skin, moisturizing.

Polyhydroxy acids: Considered one of the mildest formulations because they are larger molecules so are limited in the way they can penetrate the skin.
Uses: Softening thick, rough skin, moisturizing.

for a deep exfoliation. Follow your program daily, or twice a day if your skin can tolerate it, to avoid the buildup of keratin and dead cells, and to help moisturizers penetrate more deeply.

When trying a new skin-care product, use it regularly for at least a month before evaluating its effectiveness. Your skin fluctuates with your monthly cycle. In order to determine whether a product works for you, you'll need to use it during each phase of that cycle. Don't try more than one new product at a time, as it will be hard to tell how your skin responds to any of them.

gimme an "A"

When you hit thirty, skin can begin to look dull. Vitamin A is still the mother of all anti-aging treatments. It is essential for normal skin development, increases skin elasticity and dermal thickening, and reverses photoaging.

Products are available to give your skin some assistance. Tretinoin isn't the only form of topical vitamin A anymore. Other forms include retinyl palmitate, retinol, and tazarotene, and more are on their way.

Tretinoin (retinoic acid): A pure form of vitamin A, it can reduce fine lines, fade age spots, clear pimples, and control rosacea. Originally prescribed for acne, Retin-A (whose active ingredient is tretinoin) has been found to do much more. It exfoliates the surface of the skin, unblocking clogged pores, and forces the cells below to regenerate more quickly. It acts as a chemical peeling agent that helps the skin renew itself more rapidly, treating and preventing photoaging. The result is smoother skin thanks to the increase of collagen and elastin fibers. To see visible improvement, you have to use it for at least a month and the improvement will last only as long as it is used. It also makes the skin more sun-sensitive, so sun protection and avoiding sunlamps is vital. It does have the potential to irritate, so if you have a reaction to it, try skipping a day, using it every two days, or just applying it to wrinkle-prone areas like crow's-feet, forehead lines, and around the lips. You can also experiment with "short contact therapy," i.e., using a thin coat and washing it off after ten minutes, so penetration is limited. The key is to start with a low concentration and work your way up until you reach the highest concentration that your skin can tolerate and use it on a regular basis. Tretinoin is used in concentrations of 0.025, 0.05, and 0.01 percent and microencapsulated forms.

Tretinoin emollient cream: This prescription cream is basically Retin-A in a moisturizing base that is ideally suited to dry, aging skin. Renova has the distinction of being the only product approved by the FDA for the treatment of wrinkles. It should be applied exactly as prescribed, usually once a day at bedtime. Do not apply more or use it more often. Your wrinkles will not go away any faster and skin may be irritated. Renova may be too rich or creamy if your skin is oily or acne-prone. Tretinoin emollient cream is available in concentrations of 0.02 and 0.05 percent.

Retinol: An over-the-counter vitamin A derivative that stimulates cell division and can reduce fine lines over time. Small amounts of retinol get converted by the skin to retinoic acid, the main ingredient in Retin-A. Retinols are not as effective as tretinoin or tazarotene on fine lines, but they can be slightly less irritating. Although you won't see results as quickly, a smaller amount of Vitamin A is better than none. Over-the-counter formulas contain as little as 0.1 percent up to a maximum of 5 percent.

Good medicine

Instructions for use:
- Before applying the cream, wash your face with mild soap.
- Pat it dry and wait twenty to thirty minutes before applying the cream.
- Use a pea-size amount to cover the face.
- Wash your hands after applying it.
- Daily use of an SPF 15 is essential.

Possible side effects:
Flaking, dryness, stinging, burning, redness, irritation.

weird science

Savvy beauty consumers are demanding exceptional quality and technological innovations from skin care preparations. The next frontier in wrinkle solutions is based on clinically proven scientific advancements that can reverse the effects of aging on the skin.

It comes as no surprise that the greatest demands are for antiaging and acne products. According to the Datamonitor Report, Cosmeceutical Trends 2002, we are searching for THE skin care panacea in a relentless quest for a lineless, clear complexion in record numbers. The cosmeceutical market is predicted to grow at a rate of 15 percent annually to reach $2.1 billion by 2005.

Topical growth factors are natural proteins that facilitate communication between damaged and healthy cells and increase the rate of new cell growth to aid in wound healing. They can reverse the photodamage and accelerate healing after cosmetic surgery and laser resurfacing. Nouricel-MD, a solution derived from bioengineered human skin, is at the forefront of this new technology. It contains key growth factors cited for skin rejuvenation, including Transforming Growth Factor (TGF-Beta), Vascular Endothelial Growth Factor (VEGF), Interleukin-3, Interleukin-6, Hepatocyte Growth Factor (HGF), Platelet-derived Growth Factor (PDGF), as well as natural antioxidants, soluble collagens, and matrix proteins.

Hormones naturally found in the body include estrogen, progesterone, DHEA, androstenedione, and testosterone. As hormone production declines, everything dries out, especially the skin. Topical hormone creams with compounded estrogens are being studied for their ability to stimulate collagen formation, reduce lines, and smooth skin texture and tone.

wrinkle rescue

Prior to the advent of cosmeceuticals, we only had two basic choices for looking more youthful: makeup or surgery. Now, when your skin seems to be heading south, before you book a date with a scalpel, make sure you've covered all your bases.

Your age is not necessarily the deciding factor behind choosing a skin care regime. The driving force should be whatever are your main concerns. Are you plagued by lines around the eyes and mouth? (Think retinols and vitamin C.) Is your real pet peeve dry patches on your cheeks? (Go for hyaluronic acid and humectants.) Are the brown spots on your temples the real problem? (Try lightening agents like kojic acid, arbutin, and hydroquinone.) Once you've prioritized your issues, choose formulas for your skin type and add treatment products, one at a time, that address your specific concern.

Pay attention to the trends. Natural extracts are being substituted for many chemical substances, and plants and fermentation are replacing animals as ingredient sources. Delivery systems are more complex to offer triggered and controlled release of active ingredients. The development of more effective nanostructure and microparticle delivery systems will get larger molecules into the skin so they can work. Potent skin lightening agents that bleach discolorations for hard-to-treat areas and darker skin types are evolving. UVA/UVB protection sunscreen technology has become a mainstay in products from eye creams to foundations and lip care.

Expert advice: Look for proof of efficacy of new key ingredients and discontinue ineffective products. Trade up as new ingredients enter the market that are proven to work.

antioxidants

Scientists agree that some antioxidants fight off wrinkles from the inside and the outside, but exactly how much you need for them to work is up for debate.

Some antioxidants may hold the key to stimulating fibroblast activity to repair the dermal layer of the skin and fight free radicals. Combining several concentrated forms makes them work harder than they can on their own. Vitamins C and E work wonders as a team. C regenerates E after it has neutralized those pesky free radicals. The new kids on the block are silymarin (better known as extract of milk thistle), soya isoflavones, and green tea polyphenols, all powerful antioxidants that protect against UVA and UVB. Green tea can soothe sunburn, and is twenty times more powerful as an antioxidant than vitamin C.

A potent skin rejuvenation routine should incorporate AHAs and one of these fibroblast stimulating antioxidants: GHK copper peptides, L-ascorbic acid, or alpha lipoic acid. Together, these ingredients have the ability to repair and protect the skin, and prevent further damage. Copper plays an important role in collagen production, and has wound-healing properties. Minerals are also needed to activate antioxidant enzymes. Topical vitamin C has anti-inflammatory properties and acts as a sunscreen safety net, protecting skin from UV radiation. It has been shown to inhibit melanin production, which helps in lightening skin discolorations. The most widely touted form is L-ascorbic acid. Other forms include magnesium ascorbyl phosphate, ascorbyl palmitate, and C-Ester. Alpha lipoic acid is an antioxidant that has anti-inflammatory properties to help reduce UV light–induced inflammation within the skin.

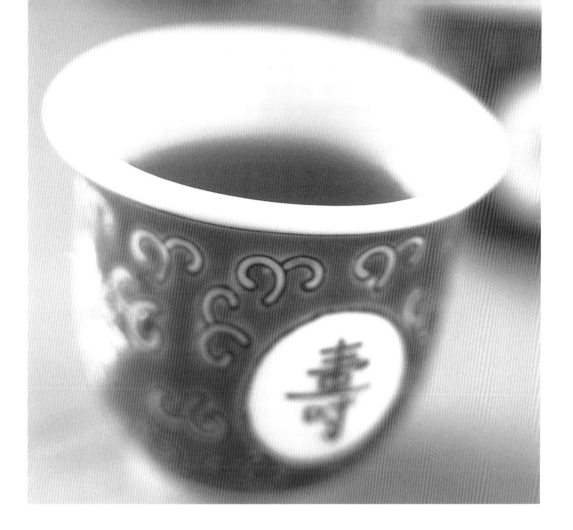

Pure antioxidants in skin care

Beta-carotene

Bioflavinoids

Blackberry extract

Blueberry extract

Coenzyme Q10 (ubiquinone)

Grape seed extract

Green tea extract

Lycopene

Marine complexes/algae

Pine tree bark extract (pycnogenol)

Pomegranate extract

Silymarin extract/milk thistle

Vitamin E (tocopherol)

White tea extract

plant sources

Phytochemicals or plant chemicals have had a major impact on antiaging skin care. They may be the next natural antidote to maturing and withering.

Phytoestrogens

Phytoestrogens, called isoflavones, mimic the effects of the female hormone, estrogen. Important phytoestrogens are genistein, daidzein, enterolactone, and equol. Wrinkle creams may contain plant hormones— like wild yam extract, a plant source for progesterone; soy, a plant source for estrogen; and melatonin, an antioxidant hormone that naturally triggers the sleep cycle. Silymarin, or milk thistle, belongs to the same family as daisies and artichokes and is commonly taken for its antitumor properties. Chemically, they have a similar effect to estrogen on the skin, which creeps away as the years fly by, causing dryness and loss of elasticity. Using hormones on your face keeps skin hydrated, firm, and toned.

Polyphenols

Polyphenols are powerful bioflavinoids or catechins. Some, like quercetin, have anti-inflammatory and healing properties. Pycnogenol, derived from the extract of pine tree bark, is a common antiaging skin-care ingredient.

Enzymes

N6-Furfuryladenine, the chemical name for kinerase, a plant growth factor that has been compared to retinoids for its effect on the skin, is known to plump up the leaves of plants by causing the surface layer to retain water. Unlike traditional moisturizers that temporarily add moisture to soften the skin's texture, this enzyme enhances cell turnover. It has the flexibility of being incorporated into a regimen of AHAs, retinol, or vitamin C, and is especially kind to recently peeled or lifted skin. It is available in 0.1 percent concentrations by prescription and 0.05 percent concentrations over the counter.

Squalene

With extracts, essences, and oils from olives being poured into luscious skin-care formulas, this little Mediterranean fruit gets top billing. Olives are rich in squalene, which can stimulate cells and enliven dry skin. Squalene belongs to the family of phytochemicals called sterols. The leaves are a source of oleuropein, an antioxidant that destroys free radicals, the oil is rich in fatty acids and glycerides for hydration, and the tree bark is a great natural exfoliant.

Expert advice: Be careful about layering your products, which can result in irritation or product interaction that can negate their effects and sensitize your skin. Avoid using the same type of ingredient in too many of your skin care products all at once.

peel me a grape

Superficial peels basically accomplish three key things: exfoliation, moisturization, and thickening the dermis. Any acid can be made to penetrate the skin lightly or deeply.

Used with active skin care, superficial peels or microdermabrasion speed up the process of exfoliation. This approach works best for modest sun damage, early wrinkling, or just plain dull-looking skin. Peels also work for precancerous actinic keratoses, hyperpigmentation, and acne scarring. Full-face chemical peels remove an entire layer of skin at once.

Low concentrations of acid produce a superficial peel; high doses are used for deeper exfoliations. The basic principle is: the deeper the peel, the better the result, the worse you look immediately afterward, and the longer it takes to heal. The other critical variable is the person who is doing the peeling and no peels are entirely idiot-proof. The word "peel" is an umbrella term used to cover a wide range of treatments starting at the level of an over-the-counter mild glycolic wash, all the way up to carbon dioxide laser resurfacing. Find out what acid is being applied and educate yourself about the various factors that affect the peel result: depth, concentration, how it is neutralized, length of time it is on the skin, and so on. Peels can be adapted to various levels depending on your needs. Apart from a basic skin classification (light to dark and tendency to burn or tan), the other factors in deciding to have a superficial peel or a deeper version are lifestyle related.

Microdermabraders are popular peel alternatives and peel boosters. Having a light microdermabrasion treatment, followed by an enzyme or acid peel, allows the solution to penetrate deeper.

Trichloracetic acid (TCA) peels (Obagi and other brands) can penetrate deeper into the skin and remove the outer layers. These peels are thought to reconstitute the lower collagen and elastin layers of the skin. There is moderate swelling of the treated areas for about a week, and scabbing will occur. Deeper peels with more concentrated solutions may take up to two weeks to heal. TCA peels are good for fine wrinkles, mild scarring, age spots, and to counteract sun damage and uneven pigmentation. Phenol peels and croton oil peels are experiencing a resurgence, and newer formulas are more buffered, with less chance of skin whitening.

Any skin type is a candidate for some form of peeling, but the darker your skin, the fewer safe peeling options you have. The deeper the peel, the greater the risk of it giving a bleaching effect (hyperpigmentation), a line of demarcation, or scarring.

WARNING: DO NOT have any peel if you are taking Accutane or if you have herpes simplex or other open lesions. If you have a history of cold sores, ask your doctor for an antiviral if having a peel or lasering around the mouth.

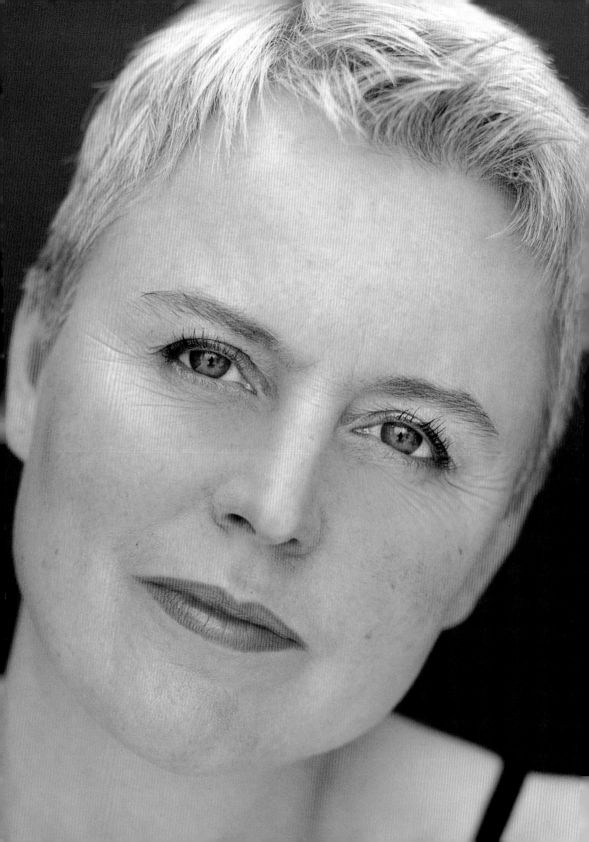

ZAPPING THEM

ZAPPING THEM

Topical skin-care products can only do so much to improve the appearance of the skin. If you want to see more dramatic improvements, you have to look to deeper remedies, the kind of treatments performed by cosmetic surgeons, dermatologists, nurses, and medical aestheticians. Today there is a wide choice of facial rejuvenation techniques, making it possible to tailor therapies to your exact needs. A variety of resurfacing methods are used to remove the topmost layers of the skin, revealing clear, unblemished skin below.

Resurfacing with lasers has traditionally involved ablative procedures that necessitated long recovery procedures and left patients red-faced for weeks or months. Although these techniques work, they are riskier and messier than many of us are willing to put up with. The newer nonablative techniques can deliver collagen remodeling that works on your wrinkles in a kinder, gentler way.

The future of skin resurfacing rests with even more high-tech light devices that can produce skin remodeling without using heat. These light-emitting sources can be used to reduce wrinkles by stimulating new collagen to fill in the lines. Stay tuned.

laser resurfacing

Laser resurfacing can remove wrinkles and red veins, lighten discolorations and age spots, and smooth scars, as well as stimulate fibroblasts to increase collagen production.

A laser is a high-energy beam of light that selectively directs its energy into tissue. It works like a scalpel that allows the doctor greater control and finesse. It applies the principles of radiation physics to narrowly segregate light of a selected wavelength and "pump" the light radiation to high intensity. The beams are targeted to a specific spot and are varied in intensity and in the duration of emitted pulses depending on their mission. Lasers and light sources are the modern way to pulverize wrinkles and extract redness from the skin. They have virtually left many older techniques in the dust.

Resurfacing with a laser should only be performed by a medical doctor. It can be done under local anesthetic with or without intravenous sedation, or a topical anesthetic cream or spray can be used for more superficial procedures. Depending on the extent of the treatment, the work can take anywhere from a few minutes to more than an hour. The laser is passed over parts of the face, neck, chest, or hands, and evaporates the surface layers of the targeted areas of skin. A new layer of pink skin is revealed. Generally, the more passes with the laser and the deeper the setting, the more extensive the treatment and longer the recovery.

The newest lasers penetrate through to the layers beneath to boost collagen production, giving skin a plumper, tighter appearance. Treatments improve skin texture and tone by stimulating new collagen in the skin to smooth it out from underneath the surface. These treatments do not destroy outer tissue as they stimulate collagen growth in the dermis, so they are safe to use on most skin types. The process is gradual and the softening of wrinkles occurs over time. You will need multiple treatment sessions in order to see results. No pain, no gain. Don't expect to be wrinkle-free at the end of one course. The advantage is zero recovery time and you won't be red for months.

The main challenges faced by lasers focus on risks versus benefits, and their safety when used on dark skin types. The darker the skin color, the more risk of lightening, darkening, or scarring from resurfacing treatments. If you have freckles on parts of your face, deeper laser resurfacing performed on one regional area like around the mouth, the lower eyelid area, or the forehead, instead of the full face, may leave you with an uneven appearance. Although the lighter lasers are not able to eradicate wrinkles and brown spots as well, they are more appealing to women who are unwilling or unable to put up with a long recovery. Nonablative techniques are good for anyone who can't take the time out for deeper procedures, or who can't commit to staying out of the sun. For extensive sun damage, different wavelengths are required.

Electrosurgical resurfacing uses coblation, a microelectrical radio frequency. Coblation delivers a pulse of energy instead of heat, to the surface of the skin. It seals blood vessels as it removes tissue and promotes skin tightening as a laser would, but by a dramatically cooler process. Electrosurgical resurfacing is good for most skin types, and the swelling and redness usually clears in two to four weeks. It can be used to improve superficial to moderate skin damage and is generally a less expensive alternative with slightly faster healing than some lasers, but the benefits may not last as long.

TOP TIP:
Laser treatments should be done under the supervision of a medical doctor who is properly trained in laser surgery. All lasers can be dangerous in the wrong hands.

laser toning

Although noninvasive resurfacing offers a lower degree of collagen remodeling than more invasive approaches do, lunchtime treatments are definitely what women want.

Nonablative systems deliver controlled energy to the skin in slightly different ways, but their mission is basically the same. The "N-Lite" Laser Collagen Replenishment System, FDA-cleared for the reduction of wrinkles around the eyes, uses a specific frequency of yellow laser light to gently stimulate growth of your body's own collagen layer. As new collagen forms, it begins to fill in the wrinkles, therefore reducing surface lines. Protective goggles are worn during the fifteen-minute treatment, and most women experience a mild tingling or slight redness, but can wear makeup right away. Any visible reduction in wrinkles requires at least a month to appear and may continue to improve for up to three months. The newly formed collagen will then age at the normal rate and the procedure is repeated for maintenance as needed. The sister treatments are called "near infrared wavelengths," ND:Yag lasers. This technology, like the CoolTouch, heats the water in the upper dermis to create a thermal wound using a cooling cryogen spray to protect the epidermis from damage. The body's response is to produce new collagen.

Intense pulsed light sources work by creating a wound in the small blood vessels in the dermis that causes collagen and vessels under the top layer to constrict. These treatments are done in a series of three-week intervals. There may be some minor discomfort, often described as similar to a rubber band snapping against the skin. A topical cream can be applied before treatment and there will be some redness and swelling that may last for one to five days. The visible reduction of fine lines and wrinkles occurs gradually over the next few weeks or months. This treatment is good for fine lines—particularly around the eyes and mouth, shallow acne scars, age spots, spider veins, rosacea, sun damage, large pores, and dark circles around the eyes.

Ablative lasers: This technology causes a burn, which removes the upper layers of skin to promote the growth of new pink skin underneath. These high-tech tools focus laser energy on damaged surface layers of skin and vaporize them, which allows a fresh layer to emerge and stimulates fibroblasts. Because of the laser beam's precision, the doctor can make several passes over areas that require extra attention without harm to adjacent skin. The two most frequently used deep lasers for skin resurfacing are carbon dioxide and Erbium:YAG.

Nonablative lasers: These laser and light sources are proving a gentle alternative for the laser phobic. The newcomers in the rapidly changing laser universe work by stimulating new collagen in the dermis, called subsurface remodeling. They essentially treat wrinkles from the inside out, rather than removing them from the outside. The laser's heat bypasses the epidermis and encourages fibroblast production, thickening the underlying collagen structure. The process of softening wrinkles continues over time as the rejuvenated skin fibers reach the surface. Procedures are repeated every four to six weeks over a six-month period to maximize new collagen formation. This technology is safer and faster than the ablative laser, recovery time is shorter, and there is less risk of pigment changes and little or no discomfort.

BEAUTY BYTES:
To find out more about lasers, log on to
www.wrinklereduction.com.

high beams

Ablative laser resurfacing is not a casual undertaking. Doctors love the effects of carbon dioxide laser treatments, but the downside is the prolonged healing and redness.

Carbon dioxide lasers: Pulsed carbon dioxide laser skin resurfacing is the gold standard for removing thin layers of skin with minimal heat damage. The laser energy is delivered to the skin at the point where superficial tissue is vaporized and destroyed and dermal damage causes collagen remodeling and skin contraction. CO_2 lasers can reach deep wrinkles, but this is a serious treatment with a long recovery period. CO_2 is still considered the workhorse of lasers because of its dramatic results on deep wrinkles, scarring, and sun damage. Typically, you will be required to apply an occlusive ointment that water cannot penetrate, for seven to ten days. The epidermis regenerates at that point, but the skin takes several weeks, up to three months, to return to normal. The fairer your skin, the longer you will stay pink. CO_2 lasers are not recommended for dark complexions because they can alter the pigment in the skin, leaving it darker or lighter.

BEAUTY BYTES:

To find out more about lasers, visit www.asds-net.org, www.aslms.org, and www.surgery.org.

Erbium YAG lasers: Erbium:YAG technology emits energy in the mid-infrared invisible light spectrum and is considered a second cousin to CO_2. Unlike CO_2 lasers, Er:YAGs produce little thermal effect. They target the skin itself and the wavelengths are absorbed by the water. Since most of our cells are predominantly water, they get absorbed by the first cells they touch. The heat effects of the laser are scattered so that thin layers of tissue can be removed with precision while minimizing damage to surrounding skin. Erbium is used for sculpting deep lines that remain after CO_2 resurfacing, and for fine lines, mild sun damage, and superficial scars. Treatment can be repeated if needed. Longer pulsed Erbium lasers deliver results that fall somewhere between CO_2 and traditional Erbium. They provide more wrinkle relief than Erbium alone, with less risk of scarring than the CO_2. Lighter ablative models, like the variable-pulsed Erbium, are also popular because they are safer for dark skin types. Combining Erbium with CO_2 can produce better results and speed up the long healing process that is associated with other lasers. Deep lasers are being used more superficially so that you can look good after a week and the pinkness fades quickly. These treatments are good for mild to moderate skin damage.

The aftermath

The big drawback of ablative lasers is the one to two weeks of postoperative care. After the skin has been treated, it is covered with either a thin film of ointment or cream, or a light synthetic breathable dressing to protect the new skin as it heals. Expect some redness, oozing, swelling, itching, and discomfort. It is critical that you follow your doctor's instructions on the proper after-care. Applying ice packs can reduce swelling and relieve discomfort for the first two days, but you will be instructed not to get the area wet. You may have to drink through a straw after treatments around the mouth area. Absolutely NO sun exposure will be allowed for at least six to eight weeks.

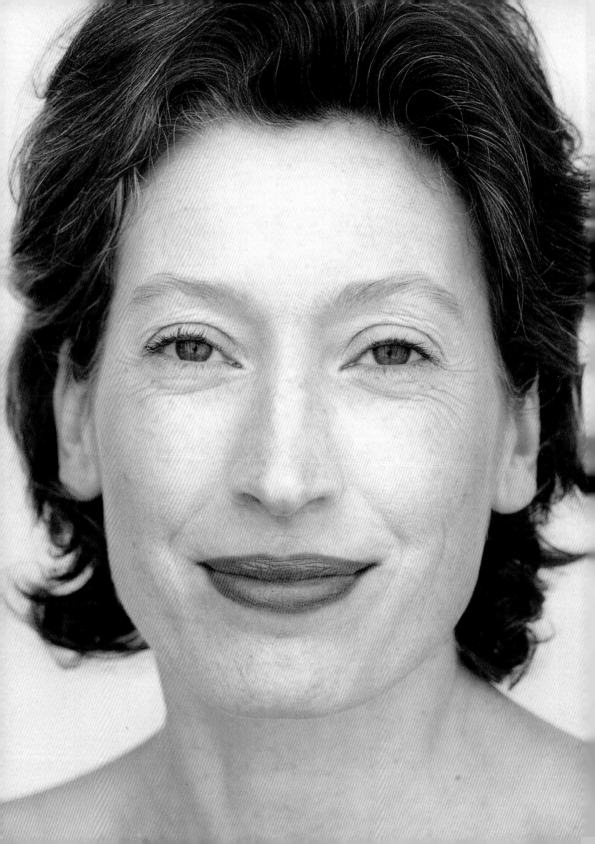

NEEDLE POINTS

There comes a point in every woman's life when all the creams, peels, and lasers together aren't enough to plump up lines, creases, and canyons. That's the time to look to wrinkle fillers. It doesn't mean you should stop all your other treatments. Fillers are just another method to add to your maintenance program. All of the minimally invasive treatments described in this book complement each other. Think of wrinkle remedies like a menu in a Chinese restaurant. Take a bit from each column to put together your perfect rejuvenation menu, and add to it as the lines get deeper. The best method is an integrated approach that may begin with one or a combination of parasurgical treatments. It's never too early to start formulating a plan for your wrinkle future, or too late.

Botulinum toxin has become the cornerstone of any antiaging program for the face. No other single product has revolutionized cosmetic medicine so much in such a relatively short time. According to the American Society for Aesthetic Plastic Surgery, in 2001, 1.6 million Botox injections were performed. It is rare to find any Botox candidate who hasn't been positively thrilled with the results. It also gives the best bang for the buck.

beauty of Botox

Botox has proved to be a little poison with unlimited health and beauty potential. A few precious drops can manage everything from frown lines, worry lines, upper lip creases, and neck cords, to excessive sweating and migraines.

After getting over the idea of having poison injected into their faces, most women get hooked. Just one treatment brings a noticeable improvement and softening of facial lines. There is literally no age that is too soon to start, and women in their late twenties and thirties are into botulinum toxin in a big way as part of an early battle against aging. Unlike fillers that plump up creases temporarily, Botox slows down the formation of new facial lines and smooths the lines already there.

New uses are discovered frequently, as doctors are becoming more experimental with its potent effects.

Where it works

Vertical lines between the brows

Lines at the bridge of the nose

Crow's-feet or squint lines

Horizontal forehead lines

Muscle bands on the neck

Under eyelid creases, muscle rolls

Décolleté lines

Chin creases and dimples

Drooping corners of the mouth

Upper and lower lip lines

How it works

The toxin acts on the junctions between nerves and muscles, preventing the release of a chemical messenger, acetylcholine, from the nerve endings. Tiny amounts are injected into a specific facial muscle so only the targeted impulse of that muscle will be blocked, immobilizing the underlying cause of the unwanted lines—muscle contractions—and prevent lines and wrinkles. Since the muscle can no longer make the offending facial expression, the lines gradually smooth out from disuse and new creases are prevented from forming. Untreated muscles are not affected, so a natural look and expressions are maintained. Some areas are less suited to this procedure because the muscles are needed for expression and important functions like eating, kissing, and opening the eyes. The goal is a softening of dynamic facial lines that won't necessarily betray your wrinkle-reducing secret. There are various strains of botulinum toxin. Type A is the most potent and commonly used.

Botulinum toxin type A: Pioneered by an ophthalmologist in 1987, its wide range of cosmetic uses has made it a mainstay in the cosmetic surgeon's arsenal of weapons for mass destruction of facial wrinkles. It received approval for cosmetic use in the United States in 2002 and is available under the trade name Botox Cosmetic by Allergan Inc., and Dysport, manufactured by Ipsen Ltd.

Botulinum toxin type B: Marketed under the name MYOBLOC in the United States and made by Elan Pharmaceuticals, it is approved for use in the treatment of cervical dystonia, a neurological disorder, and not yet approved for cosmetic uses. This form comes as a premade liquid that does not require a diluting agent, and is typically preserved in normal saline. Compared with Type A, it has a longer shelf life of up to two years and works slightly faster but is also slightly more painful when injected.

frozen assets

- Have your first treatment with someone who comes highly recommended and has a lot of experience, so that in the future you will know what is acceptable.

- Start small with one area, typically the lines between the brows or crow's-feet. Once you see the results, you can decide to have more areas worked on at your next treatment.

- If you are squeamish about needles, ask your doctor for a topical anesthetic cream or gel.

- To relieve the discomfort of the injections, apply an ice pack before and after treatment.

- If your treatment didn't work, you may have been given an overly diluted solution and need more, or it could have been injected into the wrong spot. It is exceedingly rare to be resistant to it.

- Take along a concealer to cover needle marks or tiny bruises right after treatment. Have your Botox treatment at least a week before any big social event.

- Plan your day around having your treatment—you should remain upright for three to four hours afterward.

- Botulinum toxin isn't the answer for all your wrinkles. It doesn't work as well on lines that are not entirely caused by muscle activity, like the nasal labial folds that are formed by a combination of muscle action and the weight of sagging skin.

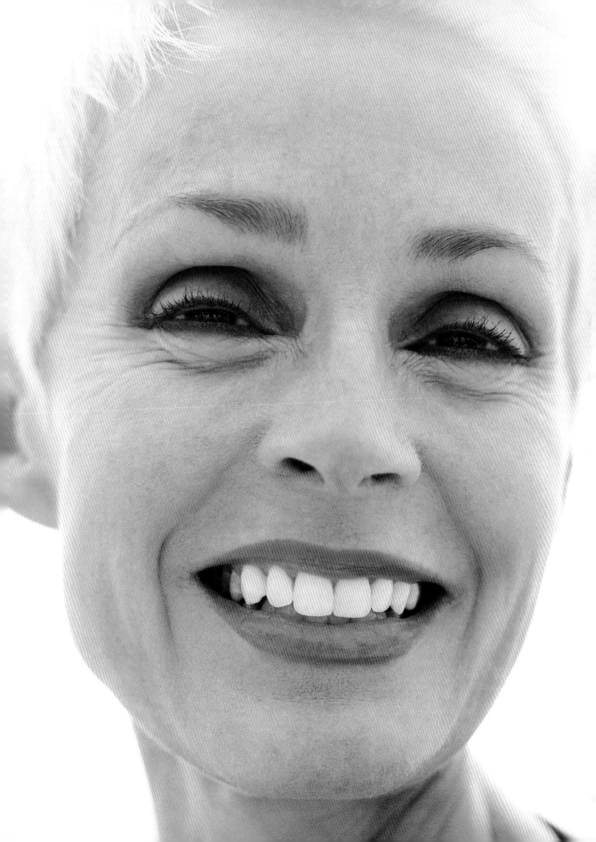

Botox budgeting

Botulinum toxin takes effect three to seven days after treatment. The improvement generally lasts for three to four months, before it gradually fades and muscle action returns.

Doctors set their fees by the area, by the treatment, or based on how much material they inject. Each area to be treated is considered a zone; for example, the crow's-feet on both sides of your face would be considered one zone; horizontal forehead lines constitute another zone; the frown lines between your eyebrows would be another zone. Each zone is usually priced separately, but most doctors discount the fee for the second and third areas. The most common combination of areas to have done in one go is: between the eyebrows, the forehead, and the crow's-feet. If you decide to do a little more for this line or that, because he is there already, don't be surprised to be charged an additional amount. Ask ahead of time what the fee will be for your treatment so you are prepared.

A single treatment will normally be sustained for up to four months, with some variation. In areas where there are two sides to be injected, as in the forehead or crow's-feet, the toxin may fade unevenly and the lines on one side return more than the lines on the other. When you begin to notice a gradual fading of its effects, you should have your next treatment. Don't wait until all of it has worn off—keep up with your treatments. When you are able to contract your facial muscles, go back for a touch-up. If you stay on top of it, you will look consistently unlined all the time. If you wait six months between treatments, until all or most of it has worn off, it will be a telltale sign that you are a Botox user. Basically, you can expect to have a treatment three to four times a year. Beware of discounted Botox—you may be paying less because you are getting less. Some doctors overdilute the solution or keep it around for too long, causing it to lose its potency. The result is that your wrinkles won't stay frozen as well or for as long. Instead of getting a good result for four months, it may only last for two, and there goes your savings!

Some people have more active muscles that require more injections, like men, and require more intense and more frequent treatments. In some cases, the more treatments you have, the longer it will last between treatments, but that is not the norm.

The real deal

Very little can go wrong with botulinum toxin, and the good news is that if it does, it is temporary. The only complications are an occasional eyelid droop, an asymmetry, or a crooked mouth. Side effects are rarely serious and always temporary, and even if you don't like the results, they are guaranteed to go away as it wears off. The problems are about technique, and some doctors are just simply better than others.

You may get a slight bruise at the injection site. To avoid bruising, don't take aspirin, anti-inflammatories, or vitamin E for one week before, and avoid having treatments done while you are menstruating, when your body is more sensitive. Some people get a slight headache that can last for a few days. After treatment, you will be instructed to smile and frown a lot for two to three hours, not to massage the area, and remain vertical for three to four hours, so it stays where it was injected and doesn't move. You should try to go back for a touch-up in two to three weeks in case any fine-tuning is needed. If too much is injected or if it is done incorrectly, the toxin can travel to nearby muscles and cause curious expressions or uneven brows.

filling station

For over a century, human-derived tissues have been used as wrinkle fillers. Today there is a wide range of biologic substances including fat, dermis, fascia, and skin, and the sources can be your own body, human, animal, as well as bioengineered.

The plumping of lines using our own tissue is vastly popular. Fat is taken from buttocks, hips, or thighs and reinjected into the necessary areas. The process involves three phases: harvesting, storing for future use, and injecting. It takes longer to perform than injecting an off-the-shelf filler, and variables include how the fat is extracted, where it is injected, how deeply, and how much. It isn't a one-time event. Fat grafting is performed under a local anesthetic and can take from thirty minutes to a few hours, depending on the extent of the work. Much of the face is suitable for transplants—the lips, nasal labial folds, and cheek hollows are among the most common.

Fat transfer is often the first choice for volume filling. Like all injectables, fat lasts better in static lines than in mobile areas such as the mouth. It is widely accepted as a stand-alone procedure, or in combination with surgery, Botox, and resurfacing.

When cosmetic surgeons assess your body, they focus on areas that are too full as well as areas that may be fat deficient, such as the buttocks in some women. In order to achieve an ideal curve, a cosmetic surgeon might need to remove fat from one area and add it to a neighboring one in order to create an ideal silhouette. The thing to remember about fat is that you usually don't have enough where you need it and almost always have too much where you don't. It is all about proportions.

One of the first signs of aging is the loss of the soft, round, cherubic fullness. By suctioning off minibits of fat, if your skin has good elasticity, it will shrink nicely and give you an improved neck contour. It's a great way to forestall a face-lift, and works well if your chin is weak or if you were born with a thick, fat neck. It doesn't always work after the mid-forties because skin shrinkage cannot be guaranteed. Women with thicker skin have a better chance of skin contraction, as do men.

Filling in the lines

As the natural fat of your face changes shape, hollows start to show up around the eyelids, the middle of the cheeks, and around the mouth. An aging face often appears more square, bottom-heavy, and angular, as soft tissue slips down from bony structures. It is not uncommon to wonder where your cheekbones have gone and notice that your jawline has lost its sharp, clean angle.

Facial fat doesn't always need to be removed, it often gets redistributed. Putting fullness back into hollows and sunken areas softens the changes associated with aging. Fat works best as a volume filler for deeper creases and folds, not fine lines. Donor fat (we've all got some of that) is taken with a small cannula or sterile tube from hips or thighs, processed to remove any blood or serum, and then reinjected into the areas to be filled. When done in stages, it allows for a gradual improvement over time without a long recovery.

The future of fat as a filler lies in stem-cell technology. You can now send your own fat to be banked for a time you might need it. Stem cells can also be harvested from fat for the purposes of growing new tissues in a lab to be reimplanted into your own body at some future date.

long shots

A face-lift doesn't get rid of wrinkles. Lasers don't fill up folds. When wrinkles deepen into folds and creases, they need to be plumped up.

Facial rejuvenation by the needle instead of the knife is big business. You would think anything that can fit into a syringe can be injected into wrinkles. Fillers can be broken down into two basic categories: resorbable and nonresorbable. The list opposite is only a partial table of the most commonly-used products.

Resorbable

Resorbable fillers are made from natural or synthetic materials that are broken down and resorbed by the body over time. They are temporary and will need to be repeated, typically in three to nine months on average. The good news is that if you are not happy with the results, it will eventually disappear. You can have other fillers injected into the same area later on. Of these, hyaluronic acid is gaining recognition as the most promising.

Nonresorbable

This class of fillers has synthetic components that don't get broken down by the body. They are considered "permanent" because the particles cannot be removed or "semipermanent" because the particles are suspended in a substance that does get resorbed in three to six months. The term "permanent" is somewhat misleading. As the aging process continues, you will need additional treatments down the line.

Wrinkle fillers

Type	Brand Name
Resorbable	
Animal derived	
Bovine collagen	Zyplast*, Zyderm*
Hyaluronic acid gel	Hylaform, Hylaform Plus, Hylaform Fine
Non-animal derived	
Hyaluronic acid gel	Restylane, Restylane Fine, Perlane, Juvederm, AcHyal, MacDermol
Polylactic acid	NewFill
Human tissue	Derived from human cadaveric tissue from a bank or autologous tissues from your body
Tissue banks	Fascialata—Fascian*
	Dermis—Cymetra*, AlloDerm*
	Collagen—Cosmoplast™, Cosmoderm™
Autologous cultured fibroblasts	Isolagen, Autologistic Tissue Injection
Nonresorbable	
Permanent	
Liquid silicone	Silikon 1000, SilSkin
Semipermanent	
Bovine collagen PMMA particles	ArteColl
Hyaluronic acid acrylic hydrogel	Dermalive

This is a partial list, including just the fillers most commonly used in the United States. Trade names vary depending on the country or region. Brand names suffixed with an asterisk indicate current FDA approval for use for facial wrinkles.

between the lines

Wrinkle fillers are like buses. A new one comes along every thirty minutes. It takes a long time to establish the long-term safety of new formulas, and no one wants to be a guinea pig.

New fillers are always under clinical investigation, and products with a high incidence of complications have difficulty getting approval in the United States, where they fall under the domain of the FDA, which has stringent requirements.

Doctors need time to determine the advantages and/or disadvantages of any new product in comparison to existing fillers on the market. The safest wrinkle-filler treatments are generally those that have the longest and best track record, meaning more people have had treatments successfully. Some women won't accept the idea of having an unknown material injected into their faces.

Only medical doctors and registered nurses (under the supervision of a medical doctor) are licensed to administer injections. Be careful about using a technician whose qualifications you are not sure of. Keep records of what treatment you had and when you had it, what worked and what caused problems. When in doubt, stick with natural fillers that are biodegradable.

Wrinkle fillers are quite variable. They can be used both as a precursor to face-lifts, as well as an alternative for the scalpel-shy, and as an addition to a surgical procedure.

filler questions

Questions to ask your doctor

- What is the source of the material?

- Is it natural or synthetic?

- What is the name of the manufacturer and where are they located? (Ask to see a product brochure.)

- How long has the filler been on the market?

- What kinds of clinical studies have been carried out on the filler?

- Is it FDA-approved?

- How long has the doctor/nurse been using it?

- What are the possible side effects?

- Do I need a skin test before treatment?

- Could I be allergic to the filler?

- What does a reaction look like and how long does it last?

- What can be done if I have a reaction to it?

- What are the risks?

- How many treatments will I need and how often?

- How much will each treatment cost?

- If it doesn't look right, what can be done to remove it?

- Can I still have other fillers later on?

choosing a surgeon

choosing a surgeon

Before going forward with any procedure, consult with at least three surgeons to get educated. Check out websites, research credentials, and insist on board certification in an appropriate speciality. If you are having surgery done in an outpatient setting, make sure the facility is fully accredited. Find the best doctors possible for whatever procedure you are considering.

General questions to ask before any surgery

What can I reasonably expect as a final result from this procedure? If appropriate, ask to meet a patient who the surgeon has recently finished working with. Seeing the results firsthand is a good indicator of what you can expect to achieve.

What training do you have, how long have you been performing this procedure, and how many times have you performed it in the last twelve months? Ask to see photographs of other procedures that the doctor has done.

What are the risks involved with this procedure? Find out how often they occur and how they will be handled if they do.

What percentage of patients have had significant complications?

What is your policy on surgical revisions? Find out about any costs for which you may be responsible if you are not happy with the end result and require a revision.

Where will the surgery be performed?

resources

For more information on beauty battles visit Wendy Lewis's website at www.wlbeauty.com. To learn more about the technologies and therapies discussed in this book, visit these websites: www.allergan.com, www.arthrocare.com, www.botox.com, www.clzr.com, www.cooltouch.com, www.elan.com, www.icnbiomed.com, www.inamed.com, www.isolagen.com, www.kinerase.com, www.laserscope.com, www.lpgone.net, www.lumenis.com, www.new-fill.com, www.obagi.com, www.orthodermatological.com, www.procyte.com, www.qmed-aesthetics.com, www.sciton.com, www.skinmedica.com, www.stellsource.com, www.sunandskin.com, www.thermage.com, www.triluma.com, and www.wrinklereduction.com.

acknowledgments

The author wishes to thank the following physicians and specialists for sharing their expertise for this book: Fredric Brandt, MD; Harold Brody, MD; Lisa Donofrio, MD; Steven Fagien, MD; Peter Bela Fodor, MD; Bryan Forley, MD; Oz Garcia; Ellen Gendler, MD; Roy Geronemus, MD; David J. Goldberg, MD; Mitchel Goldman, MD; Arielle Kauvar, MD; Laurence Kirwan, MD; Albert Lefkovits, MD; Lyle Leipziger, MD; Ted Lockwood, MD; Z. Paul Lorenc, MD; Alan Matarasso, MD; Seth Matarasso, MD; Roy Michaels Salon; Foad Nahai, MD; Gerald Pitman, MD; Rod Rohrich, MD; Ronald Savin, MD; Robin Unger, MD; Walter Unger, MD; Ken Washenik, MD; Frank Weiser, MD; Patricia Wexler, MD; Donald Wood-Smith, MD.

picture credits